NATIONAL ACADEMIES *Sciences Engineering Medicine*

NATIONAL ACADEMIES PRESS
Washington, DC

Mitigating Arboviral Threats and Strengthening Public Health Preparedness

Elizabeth Ashby Guo, Claire Biffl, and Robert Pool, *Rapporteurs*

Forum on Microbial Threats

Board on Global Health

Health and Medicine Division

Proceedings of a Workshop

NATIONAL ACADEMIES PRESS 500 Fifth Street, NW Washington, DC 20001

This activity was supported by contracts between the National Academy of Sciences and the American Society of Tropical Medicine and Hygiene, Burroughs Wellcome Fund (Contract No. 1195124), Centers for Disease Control and Prevention (Contract No. 75D30121D11240, Order No. 75D30122F00011), EcoHealth Alliance, Infectious Diseases Society of America, Johnson & Johnson (Contract No. C2023026615), Merck and Co., Inc. (Grant No. MEM-22-160471), National Institute of Allergy and Infectious Diseases, National Institutes of Health (Contract No. HHSN263201800029I, Task Order No. 75N98023F00023), New Venture Fund (Contract No. NVF-NGDF-NAT10-Subgrant-022263-2023-08-01), Sanofi, Society of Infectious Diseases Pharmacists, U.S. Agency for International Development (Contract No. 7200AA18GR00003), Uniformed Services University of the Health Sciences (Contract No. HU00012210001), and U.S. Department of Veterans Affairs (Contract No. 36C25024P0225). Any opinions, findings, conclusions, or recommendations expressed in this publication do not necessarily reflect the views of any organization or agency that provided support for the project.

International Standard Book Number-13: 978-0-309-71927-8
International Standard Book Number-10: 0-309-71927-5
Digital Object Identifier: https://doi.org/10.17226/27774

This publication is available from the National Academies Press, 500 Fifth Street, NW, Keck 360, Washington, DC 20001; (800) 624-6242 or (202) 334-3313; http://www.nap.edu.

Copyright 2024 by the National Academy of Sciences. National Academies of Sciences, Engineering, and Medicine and National Academies Press and the graphical logos for each are all trademarks of the National Academy of Sciences. All rights reserved.

Printed in the United States of America.

Suggested citation: National Academies of Sciences, Engineering, and Medicine. 2024. *Mitigating arboviral threats and strengthening public health preparedness: Proceedings of a workshop*. Washington, DC: The National Academies Press. https://doi.org/10.17226/27774.

The **National Academy of Sciences** was established in 1863 by an Act of Congress, signed by President Lincoln, as a private, nongovernmental institution to advise the nation on issues related to science and technology. Members are elected by their peers for outstanding contributions to research. Dr. Marcia McNutt is president.

The **National Academy of Engineering** was established in 1964 under the charter of the National Academy of Sciences to bring the practices of engineering to advising the nation. Members are elected by their peers for extraordinary contributions to engineering. Dr. John L. Anderson is president.

The **National Academy of Medicine** (formerly the Institute of Medicine) was established in 1970 under the charter of the National Academy of Sciences to advise the nation on medical and health issues. Members are elected by their peers for distinguished contributions to medicine and health. Dr. Victor J. Dzau is president.

The three Academies work together as the **National Academies of Sciences, Engineering, and Medicine** to provide independent, objective analysis and advice to the nation and conduct other activities to solve complex problems and inform public policy decisions. The National Academies also encourage education and research, recognize outstanding contributions to knowledge, and increase public understanding in matters of science, engineering, and medicine.

Learn more about the National Academies of Sciences, Engineering, and Medicine at **www.nationalacademies.org**.

Consensus Study Reports published by the National Academies of Sciences, Engineering, and Medicine document the evidence-based consensus on the study's statement of task by an authoring committee of experts. Reports typically include findings, conclusions, and recommendations based on information gathered by the committee and the committee's deliberations. Each report has been subjected to a rigorous and independent peer-review process and it represents the position of the National Academies on the statement of task.

Proceedings published by the National Academies of Sciences, Engineering, and Medicine chronicle the presentations and discussions at a workshop, symposium, or other event convened by the National Academies. The statements and opinions contained in proceedings are those of the participants and are not endorsed by other participants, the planning committee, or the National Academies.

Rapid Expert Consultations published by the National Academies of Sciences, Engineering, and Medicine are authored by subject-matter experts on narrowly focused topics that can be supported by a body of evidence. The discussions contained in rapid expert consultations are considered those of the authors and do not contain policy recommendations. Rapid expert consultations are reviewed by the institution before release.

For information about other products and activities of the National Academies, please visit www.nationalacademies.org/about/whatwedo.

PLANNING COMMITTEE ON MITIGATING ARBOVIRAL THREATS AND STRENGTHENING PUBLIC HEALTH PREPAREDNESS[1]

PETER DASZAK (*Co-Chair*), President, EcoHealth Alliance
THOMAS W. SCOTT (*Co-Chair*), Distinguished Professor Emeritus, University of California, Davis
KEVIN ANDERSON, retired, formerly U.S. Department of Homeland Security
MARCOS ESPINAL, retired, former Assistant Director, Pan American Health Organization
EVA HARRIS, Professor, University of California, Berkeley
KENT E. KESTER, Vice President, Translational Medicine, International AIDS Vaccine Initiative
ALBERT I. KO, Raj and Indra Nooyi Professor of Public Health, Yale University
LINDA S. LLOYD, Independent Consultant; Lecturer, San Diego State University
VALERIE A. PAZ-SOLDÁN, Associate Professor, Tulane University School of Public Health and Tropical Medicine
BENJAMIN PINSKY, Professor of Pathology and Medicine, Stanford University School of Medicine
ANN M. POWERS, Associate Director for Science, Centers for Disease Control and Prevention

Staff

ELIZABETH ASHBY GUO, Program Officer
CLAIRE BIFFL, Research Associate (*through July 2024*)
ERIKA CHOW, Research Assistant
SAMUEL CRAWFORD, Research Associate
NICKY KUANG, Senior Program Assistant (*through October 2023*)
JULIE LIAO, Director, Forum on Microbial Threats
JULIE PAVLIN, Science Advisor; Senior Board Director, Board on Global Health

Consultant

ROBERT POOL, Science Writer

---

[1] The National Academies of Sciences, Engineering, and Medicine's planning committees are solely responsible for organizing the workshop, identifying topics, and choosing speakers. The responsibility for the published Proceedings of a Workshop rests with the workshop rapporteurs and the institution.

FORUM ON MICROBIAL THREATS[1]

PETER DASZAK (*Chair*), President, EcoHealth Alliance
CRISTINA CASSETTI (*Vice Chair*), Deputy Director, Division of Microbial and Infectious Diseases, National Institute of Allergy and Infectious Diseases, National Institutes of Health
KENT E. KESTER (*Vice Chair*), Vice President of Translational Medicine, International AIDS Vaccine Initiative
EMILY ABRAHAM, Director, External Affairs and Policy, Global Public Health at Johnson & Johnson
KEVIN ANDERSON, retired, U.S. Department of Homeland Security
DAN H. BAROUCH, Director, Center for Virology and Vaccine Research, Beth Israel Deaconess Medical Center; William Bosworth Castle Professor of Medicine, Harvard Medical School
DANIEL BAUSCH, President, American Society of Tropical Medicine and Hygiene; Senior Director, Emerging Threats and Global Health Security, FIND
NAHID BHADELIA, Founding Director, Boston University Center for Emerging Infectious Diseases Policy and Research
CHRISTOPHER BRADEN, Principal Deputy Director, National Center for Emerging and Zoonotic Infectious Diseases, U.S. Centers for Disease Control and Prevention
RICK A. BRIGHT, Founder, Bright Global Health
AMBIKA BUMB, Deputy Executive Director, Bipartisan Commission on Biodefense
ANDREW CLEMENTS, Senior Scientific Advisor, Emerging Threats Division, U.S. Agency for International Development
GREG FRANK, Director of Global Public Policy, Merck & Co., Inc.
WONDWOSSEN GEBREYES, Executive Director of Global One Health Initiative, The Ohio State University
BRUCE G. GELLIN, Senior Vice President and Chief of Global Public Health Strategy, Rockefeller Foundation
GIGI KWIK GRONVALL, Associate Professor, Johns Hopkins University Center for Health Security
ELIZABETH D. HERMSEN, Lead, Global Antimicrobial Resistance and Antimicrobial Stewardship Medical Affairs, Pfizer
ALBERT I. KO, Raj and Indra Nooyi Professor of Public Health, Yale School of Public Health; Professor of Epidemiology and Medicine, Yale School of Medicine

---

[1] The National Academies of Sciences, Engineering, and Medicine's forums and roundtables do not issue, review, or approve individual documents. The responsibility for the published Proceedings of a Workshop rests with the workshop rapporteurs and the institution.

MARK G. KORTEPETER, Vice President for Research, Professor of Preventive Medicine and Medicine, Uniformed Services University of the Health Sciences
LINDA S. LLOYD, Independent Consultant; Lecturer, San Diego State University School of Public Health
SYRA MADAD, Senior Director, Special Pathogens Program, NYC Health + Hospitals
JONNA H. MAZET, Vice Provost—Grand Challenges, University of California, Davis
VICTORIA McGOVERN, Chief Strategy Officer and the Gertrude Elion Endowed Program Officer, Burroughs Wellcome Fund
SUMIKO MEKARU, Vice President, Research and Innovation, The Public Health Company
TIMOTHY D. MURRAY, Professor, Rosalie and Harold Rea Brown Distinguished Endowed Chair, Washington State University
MELISSA NOLAN, Associate Professor, Arnold School of Public Health, University of South Carolina
RAFAEL OBREGÓN, Country Representative, UNICEF Nicaragua
BENJAMIN PINSKY, Professor of Pathology and Medicine, Stanford University School of Medicine
AMEET J. PINTO, Associate Professor and Carlton S. Wilder Junior Faculty Chair, Georgia Institute of Technology
P. DAVID ROGERS, Chair, Department of Pharmacy and Pharmaceutical Sciences, St. Jude Children's Research Hospital
GARY A. ROSELLE, Executive Director, National Infectious Disease Services Program, Veterans Health Administration, U.S. Department of Veterans Affairs
UMAIR SHAH, Secretary of Health, Washington State
JONATHAN SLEEMAN, Senior Science Advisor, U.S. Geological Survey
MATTHEW ZAHN, Deputy Health Officer, Orange County Health Care Agency

Forum on Microbial Threats Staff

ELIZABETH ASHBY GUO, Program Officer
CLAIRE BIFFL, Research Associate (*through July 2024*)
NICKY KUANG, Senior Program Assistant (*through October 2023*)
JULIE LIAO, Director, Forum on Microbial Threats
JULIE PAVLIN, Science Advisor; Senior Board Director, Board on Global Health
TAYLOR WINDMILLER, Senior Program Assistant (*from January 2024*)

Reviewers

This Proceedings of a Workshop was reviewed in draft form by individuals chosen for their diverse perspectives and technical expertise. The purpose of this independent review is to provide candid and critical comments that will assist the National Academies of Sciences, Engineering, and Medicine in making each published proceedings as sound as possible and to ensure that it meets the institutional standards for quality, objectivity, evidence, and responsiveness to the charge. The review comments and draft manuscript remain confidential to protect the integrity of the process.

We thank the following individuals for their review of this proceedings:

KEVIN K. ARIËN, Institute of Tropical Medicine
LEAH KATZELNICK, National Institutes of Health

Although the reviewers listed above provided many constructive comments and suggestions, they were not asked to endorse the content of the proceedings nor did they see the final draft before its release. The review of this proceedings was overseen by **DAVID R. CHALLONER,** Vice President for Health Affairs (emeritus), University of Florida. He was responsible for making certain that an independent examination of this proceedings was carried out in accordance with standards of the National Academies and that all review comments were carefully considered. Responsibility for the final content rests entirely with the rapporteur and the National Academies.

We also thank staff member David Butler, the National Academy of Engineering Holloman Scholar, for reading and providing helpful comments on this manuscript.

Contents

ACRONYMS AND ABBREVIATIONS — xv

1 INTRODUCTION — 1
   Structure of the Proceedings, 3
   References, 3

2 CURRENT AND EMERGING THREATS FROM ARBOVIRAL
   DISEASES: EXISTING BURDEN AND FUTURE RISK — 5
   Advancing Global Research Priorities: Lessons from Zika, 6
   Overview of Arboviral Disease: The Current Status and Future
       of Disease Control, 11
   Country and Regional Experience: Impacts and Challenges
       of Arboviral Control, 13
   Discussion, 22
   References, 23

3 ASSESSING AND DETECTING ARBOVIRAL RISK — 25
   Epidemiological Surveillance, 26
   Genomic Surveillance, 29
   Integrated Surveillance and Risk Assessment: Case Study
       from Singapore, 33
   Diagnostics for Arbovirus Mitigation, 36
   Discussion, 39
   References, 40

4	**RESPONSE TO ARBOVIRAL THREATS**	**43**

Arbovirus Vaccines, 44
Vector Control, 49
Integrated Surveillance in the Americas, 51
Predictive Tools and Modeling, 54
Discussion, 57
References, 59

5	**LESSONS LEARNED FROM PREVIOUS OUTBREAKS**	**61**

Previous Arboviral Outbreaks, 62
COVID-19, 66
Discussion, 69
References, 72

6	**ARBOVIRUS SPILLOVER AND SPREAD**	**75**

Zoonotic Disease Spillover and Emergence, 77
Implementation Science: Operationalizing One Health Data, 79
Ranking Disease Threats, 82
Behavior Management to Prevent Spillover and Spread, 85
Discussion, 88
References, 90

7	**URBAN DEVELOPMENT AND MANAGEMENT**	**93**

Vision for Building *Aedes* Out, 94
Public Health in Urban Environments, 97
Case Study From Singapore, 99
Urban Mosquito Control in Africa and the New Mosquito on the Block, 102
Discussion, 105
References, 107

8	**STRENGTHENING PREPAREDNESS FOR ARBOVIRAL DISEASES**	**109**

Priorities, 109
Question-and-Answer Period, 117

9	**CLOSING REMARKS**	**119**

APPENDIXES
A Workshop Statement of Task 125
B Public Meeting Agenda 127

Figures

FIGURES

3-1 Exponential growth of genomic sequencing data for arboviral threats, 30

5-1 Number of diagnostic samples received at the CDC's Arboviral Diseases Branch diagnostics laboratory by month from January 2010–May 2016, 63

6-1 The factors in determining the risk score for each virus, 83
6-2 Weighted scores in the arbovirus risk assessment displayed in two dimensions, 84
6-3 Consolidated framework for implementation research, 86

7-1 Dengue incidence and *Aedes* population density (house index) in Singapore, 1966–2022, 100
7-2 *Anopheles stephensi* is spreading across Africa, 104

Acronyms and Abbreviations

Africa CDC	Africa Centres for Disease Control and Prevention
CDC	Centers for Disease Control and Prevention
CREATE-NEO	Coordinating Research on Emerging Arboviral Threats Encompassing the Neotropics
ELISA	enzyme-linked immunosorbent assay
FDA	Food and Drug Administration
IgG	immunoglobulin G
IgM	immunoglobulin M
mRNA	messenger RNA
NAAT	nucleic acid amplification tests
NIH	National Institutes of Health
NS1	non-structural protein 1 (used in dengue virus diagnostic test)
PAHO	Pan American Health Organization
PCR	polymerase chain reaction
PLISA	Health Information Platform for the Americas
RCT	randomized controlled trial

RDT	rapid diagnostic test
RNA	ribonucleic acid
RT-PCR	reverse transcription–polymerase chain reaction
UN	United Nations
UNICEF	United Nations Children's Fund
USAID	U.S. Agency for International Development
WHO	World Health Organization

1

Introduction

Arboviruses, or viruses carried by arthropods such as mosquitoes or ticks (arthropod-borne viruses), are responsible for an estimated 700,000 deaths worldwide each year (Byaruhanga et al., 2023). With the changing global climate, the geographic distribution of these diseases, which include Zika, dengue, chikungunya, West Nile, and yellow fever, are steadily expanding. At the time of this workshop, half of the world's population—about 4 billion people—are at risk of infection by dengue, a potentially fatal disease in its severe form (Brady et al., 2012; Madewell, 2020; WHO, 2023). To address this growing threat and the impact of global climate change, the Forum on Microbial Threats of the National Academies of Sciences, Engineering, and Medicine convened experts from medical entomology; local, state, and federal public health; ecology; arbovirology; immunology; disease modeling; and urban planning at a public workshop in Washington, DC, on December 12–13, 2023, to explore avenues of threat reduction from known and emerging arboviral diseases with a focus on building long-term public health resilience. This proceedings is developed from the presentations and discussions at the workshop, titled Mitigating Arboviral Threats and Strengthening Public Health Preparedness.[1]

---

[1] The planning committee's role was limited to planning the workshop, and the workshop summary has been prepared by the workshop rapporteurs as a factual summary of what occurred at the workshop. Statements, recommendations, and opinions expressed are those of individual presenters and participants and are not necessarily endorsed or verified by the National Academies of Sciences, Engineering, and Medicine, and they should not be construed as reflecting any group consensus.

As workshop co-chair Thomas W. Scott of the University of California, Davis, presented in his opening remarks, arboviruses are a particularly difficult public health issue to address because of their complex transmission cycles. The presence of a vector host, such as a mosquito, in disease transmission complicates infection prevention measures because the vector organism has its independent ecology, population structure, genetics, and unique biological interactions with the virus. In some cases, there can be multiple vectors that are capable of infecting humans with the virus. Additional layers of complexity are introduced when non-human animals are part of the pathogen life cycle.[2] Either domesticated or wild animals can serve as reservoirs for these viruses, and as sources of unpredictable disease spillovers into human populations.

Despite these complexities and the challenges they present in identifying and implementing effective control strategies for arboviral diseases, Scott said, the workshop planning committee saw opportunities in achieving major public health advances to alleviate the vast toll of these diseases. Attributing this hope to tremendous advances in the field he observed in the past decade, Scott explained, "I've been working on arboviruses for about 47 years, and in the last 10 years I've seen the most innovation in the field of any time in my career."

To further explore those advancements and remaining challenges, the Forum on Microbial Threats held the public workshop, Mitigating Arboviral Threats and Strengthening Public Health Preparedness,[3] with the primary goal of highlighting promising scientific breakthroughs that can be translated into improved public health actions. The forum has held two prior workshops related to arboviruses. The first, held in 2007, sought to clarify the environments, human health, and ecological connections in the emergence and spread of vector-borne diseases (IOM, 2008). The second, held in 2014, examined the global health impacts of vector-borne diseases (NASEM, 2016). Scott pointed out that a central charge for this planning committee was to consider "how can we do things differently, in a sustainable way, to prevent arboviral diseases" in the face of the growing geographical distribution of arboviruses and the toll of these diseases. The aim of the workshop was to explore the role of arbovirus mitigation within the context of public health preparedness and capacity building.

---

[2] One example is the transmission of Lyme disease, where the arthropod vector (black-legged tick) carrying the disease-causing bacteria can feed and proliferate on a wide range of non-human vertebrate hosts including birds, lizards, and other mammals that contribute to a persistent pathogen reservoir. See https://www.ncbi.nlm.nih.gov/pmc/articles/PMC5879012/ (accessed June 30, 2024).

[3] Video recordings of this workshop and all slide decks used by speakers are available on the Forum on Microbial Threats' webpage. https://www.nationalacademies.org/event/40925_12-2023_mitigating-arboviral-threats-and-strengthening-public-health-preparedness-a-workshop (accessed July 1, 2024).

Discussion focused on potential actions that can be taken to understand and mitigate arboviral disease threats and highlight priority areas for research and investment.[4]

STRUCTURE OF THE PROCEEDINGS

The workshop's first day centered on the current landscape of arboviral threats and factors in assessing their risks to human health. Chapter 1 summarizes introductory remarks that explain the context and rationale for convening this workshop. Chapter 2 provides an overview of global arbovirus research priorities as well as current and emerging arboviral disease threats, noting in particular the knowledge gaps and key challenges. Chapter 3 covers topics of detecting and assessing arboviral risks to guide and evaluate various intervention strategies. Chapter 4 is devoted to various responses to arboviral threats, including surveillance, vector control, vaccines, and predictive tools. Chapter 5 delves into lessons learned from previous outbreaks of arboviruses and from the COVID-19 pandemic, and how these lessons might guide future responses.

The second day of the workshop centered on innovations for future arboviral disease mitigation. Chapter 6 examines the spillover and spread of arboviruses and how this knowledge may inform interventions. Chapter 7 focuses on urban development and how constructing and managing urban environments could have a sustainable impact on arboviral infections. Chapter 8 captures reflections from workshop speakers who highlighted ideas from the workshop that they found to be the most consequential in strengthening preparedness for future arboviral disease outbreaks. A short synthesis of the workshop's key themes from Scott at the close of the workshop is presented in Chapter 9.

REFERENCES

Brady, O. J., P. W. Gething, S. Bhatt, J. P. Messina, J. S. Brownstein, A. G. Hoen, C. L. Moyes, A. W. Farlow, T. W. Scott, and S. I. Hay. 2012. Refining the global spatial limits of dengue virus transmission by evidence-based consensus. *PLOS Neglected Tropical Diseases* 6(8):e1760.

Byaruhanga, T., J. T. Kayiwa, A. M. Nankya, I. J. Ataliba, C. P. McClure, J. K. Bell, and J. J. Lutwama. 2023. Arbovirus circulation, epidemiology, and spatiotemporal distribution in Uganda. *IJID Regions* 6:171–176.

IOM (Institute of Medicine). 2008. *Vector-Borne Diseases: Understanding the Environmental, Human Health, and Ecological Connections: Workshop Summary.* Washington, DC: National Academy Press.

---

[4] The full Statement of Task is provided in Appendix A. The workshop agenda is provided in Appendix B.

Madewell, Z. J. 2020. Arboviruses and their vectors. *Southern Medical Journal* 113(10):520–523.
NASEM (National Academies of Sciences, Engineering, and Medicine). 2016. *Global Health Impacts of Vector-Borne Diseases: Workshop Summary*. Washington, DC: The National Academies Press.
WHO (World Health Organization). 2023. Dengue and severe dengue. https://www.who.int/news-room/fact-sheets/detail/dengue-and-severe-dengue (accessed March 13, 2024).

2

Current and Emerging Threats from Arboviral Diseases: Existing Burden and Future Risk

---

Highlights

- In recent decades there has been a global resurgence in emergent arbovirus outbreaks for various reasons, including increased urbanization and the rise of megacities, increased population mobility, and a decline in the necessary public health infrastructure. (Gubler, Velayudhan)
- Reversing the trend of emergent arboviral diseases will require getting serious about prevention; coordinating global funding to help those countries most at risk; the development of operational and response plans with automatic triggers, laboratory-based proactive surveillance, and urban renewal; and increased research into vector control, vaccines, therapeutics, diagnostics, insecticides, and surveillance. (Gubler, Velayudhan)
- The region of the Americas presents a constant circulation of emerging and reemerging arboviruses, many of which have high epidemic potential, and this is a permanent risk to public health. (Aldighieri)
- Even as the case numbers of diseases like dengue increase, countries can reduce the proportion of cases that progress to severe disease and death through systematic capacity-building efforts. (Aldighieri)
- Climate change is increasing the suitability of the environment for *Aedes aegypti* at a growing rate. (Aldighieri)

continued

- The United States has multiple endemic mosquito-borne viruses and has seen several outbreaks of viruses introduced from outside the country. (Kramer)
- Vector control can be complicated by the presence of different vectors with various distributions and behaviors. (Kramer)
- Challenges to the control of arboviral diseases include insufficient multisectoral coordination of responses; the need for capacity building in clinical, entomological, and vector control staff; the difficulties of clinical diagnosis; and limited laboratory capacity and inadequate supplies. (Velayudhan)
- The One Health approach is the most effective way to deal with arbovirus threats. (Kramer)

NOTE: These points were made by the individual workshop speakers/participants identified above. They are not intended to reflect a consensus among workshop participants.

The workshop opened with an overview from Eve Lackritz, the deputy director of the Center for Infectious Disease Research and Policy at the University of Minnesota, of efforts that have been dedicated to respond to Zika virus outbreaks, triggered by the 2014–2016 epidemic that emerged in Brazil. This was followed by a panel of speakers that discussed the threats, current and future, posed by arboviruses around the world.

ADVANCING GLOBAL RESEARCH PRIORITIES: LESSONS FROM ZIKA

Lackritz illustrated the range of challenges in mitigating arboviral threats by focusing on the experience with the Zika virus. Drawing from a recent international meeting on Zika and mosquito-borne arboviruses, her remarks reflect efforts over the past several years to develop strategic priorities to advance research and development of diagnostics, vaccines, and therapeutics to counter these pathogens.

Spread mainly by *Aedes aegypti* and *Aedes albopictus* mosquitoes, Zika rose to prominence for global health officials from the major 2015–2016 outbreak that emerged in Brazil and rapidly spread throughout the Americas (CDC, 2019). Although most cases are mild or asymptomatic, Zika can cause microcephaly, neurodevelopmental delay, and other severe congenital malformations in infants born to women who are infected during pregnancy. To date, locally acquired mosquito-borne transmission of Zika virus has been identified in more than 90 countries and territories worldwide (WHO, 2022). Lackritz observed a global sense of complacency about the virus that seems to have developed since the end of the 2016 epidemic, noting that there are still currently no approved vaccines to prevent infection, no therapeutics to treat the disease, and no diagnostics for routine screening of pregnant women. Cautioning that there is a serious possibility of a large-scale Zika outbreak reemergence, she pointed out that it is "a critical time to develop countermeasures and to figure out how to be prepared for reemergence in the future."

Research and development of medical countermeasures against Zika is particularly challenging compared with other arboviruses, Lackritz noted at the start. Main characteristics of Zika disease that contribute to its unique challenges in conducting research include: its frequency of co-circulation and co-infection with other arboviruses, its relatively low rate of transmission, uncertainty in its future transmission patterns, and the goal of preventing infection of the fetus while the disease is largely asymptomatic and undetected in adults.

First, Lackritz highlighted the need to prioritize the development of diagnostics in order to mitigate challenges in prevention and response efforts. Without diagnostics, it is difficult to carry out research, preparation, response efforts, disease forecasting, or the evaluation of public health interventions such as vector control, she said. The currently available diagnostic options each have trade-offs that preclude their broad use in outbreak settings. One diagnostic option, nucleic acid amplification tests (NAAT), have good specificity but only a very narrow window in which the viral ribonucleic acid (RNA) is detectable. NAATs thus have limited utility for identifying asymptomatic infections and for routine screenings and in antenatal care. By contrast, immunoglobulin M (IgM) may persist for up to 3 months, which provides a larger window for detection. This means that a positive IgM test might reflect an infection that occurred before pregnancy. IgM also has cross-reactivity with other flaviviruses,[1] so a positive result does not necessarily indicate a Zika infection. The plaque-reduction neutralization test is labor-intensive and limited to reference laboratories, and it often does not identify the etiologic agent due to cross-reactivity. There is also a lack of approved tests for other specimen types including urine, cerebrospinal fluid, and amniotic fluid. "There is clearly a need for rapid and simple tests," Lackritz concluded. Clinicians facing a Zika outbreak need point-of-care diagnostics that work in settings with limited lab capacity. Lackritz shared that there were multiple NAAT and serologic assays

---

[1] The genus *Flavivirus* was renamed to *Orthoflavivirus* in April 2023, though the majority of literature at this point still refer to the old nomenclature. See https://link.springer.com/article/10.1007/s00705-023-05835-1 (accessed June 30, 2024). This proceedings will use the term "flavivirus" for consistency with the speaker presentation material. For disambiguation, the proceedings will note where the speaker used "flavivirus" to refer to the family Flaviviridae instead of the genus *Flavivirus*.

approved under emergency use authorizations during the 2015 outbreak, but they were never validated by standardized evaluations.

On the current state and challenges of research and development for Zika vaccines, therapeutics, and prophylaxis, Lackritz conceded that understanding the immunology of Zika infections is difficult and further confounded by complex immunologic interactions with co-circulating flaviviruses. The potential cross-reactivity with co-circulating flaviviruses raises the concern for antibody-dependent enhancement from vaccination and underscore the need for better understanding of protective immunity. At the time of this workshop, the mechanisms by which the approved flavivirus vaccines create protective immunity remain poorly understood, so neutralizing antibodies are often used as correlates of protection. Lackritz highlighted a need to elucidate the roles of neutralizing and non-neutralizing antibodies as well as T cell–mediated immune responses in conferring protection from infection, disease development, and transmission. Another issue is that the prevention of congenital infection is an unrealistic endpoint of clinical trials as it is a relatively rare event on a population level, so it is impossible with a clinical trial to observe whether the vaccine is doing what it is designed to do. Finally, since most infections are asymptomatic, it is difficult to assess clinical endpoints and benefit for regulatory approval.

There are a number of Zika vaccine candidates based on different platforms and antigens in various stages of development at the time of the workshop, with some as far as in phase 2 clinical trials, Lackritz said.[2] However, this diversity also contributes to difficulties in interpreting clinical trial data due to a lack of standardization and points of comparison between the different methods, laboratory criteria, and trial endpoints. Another issue is the challenge of defining clinical trial endpoints. Despite its biological and epidemiological significance, prevention of congenital infection is a challenging endpoint for clinical trials as it is a relatively rare event on a population level, Lackritz said, and testing the prevention of congenital Zika infection will require a large sample size collected over many years. An additional and unique consideration in developing a Zika vaccine is the potential legal liabilities associated with its use in pregnant women or women who might become pregnant. She added that, since most infections are asymptomatic, it is also difficult to assess clinical endpoints and benefit for regulatory approval. This contributes to the uncertainty in market demand and unstable funding to developing Zika vaccines.

Several potential regulatory pathways exist to the approval of a Zika vaccine. For example, Lackritz pointed out, a chikungunya vaccine was

---

[2] For more information on Zika vaccine candidate platforms and components see Figure 1 in https://doi.org/10.1080/21645515.2020.1730657 (accessed July 1, 2024).

just approved through a combination of efficacy testing in animal models and immunogenicity testing in humans. Acknowledging that regulatory pathways differ by country, Lackritz noted that the most likely path for a Zika vaccine to receive approval by the U.S. Food and Drug Administration (FDA) would be a stepwise approach with an accelerated pathway approval for adults combined with post-marketing studies to monitor for populational immunity and the impact on fetuses. Altogether, Lackritz said, it will be necessary to clearly identify the target populations in designing clinical trials as well as nontraditional regulatory pathways that a potential Zika vaccine could take to garner approval.

One challenge in developing a Zika vaccine that Lackritz highlighted is that any agent used in pregnant women or women who might become pregnant creates various potential legal liabilities for the company developing the vaccine. Testing the prevention of congenital Zika infection will require a large sample size collected over many years. Several potential regulatory pathways exist to the approval of a Zika vaccine. For example, Lackritz pointed out, a chikungunya vaccine was just approved through a combination of efficacy testing in animal models and immunogenicity testing in humans. Acknowledging that regulatory pathways differ by country, Lackritz noted that it seems the most likely path to approval of a Zika vaccine by the U.S. FDA would be a stepwise approach with an accelerated pathway approval for adults combined with post-marketing studies to monitor for populational immunity and the impact on fetuses.

Next, Lackritz described some systematic approaches that could accelerate research and development for Zika diagnostics, vaccines, and therapeutics. First, she focused on the use of biorepositories and specimen sharing. Researchers at the recent international meeting highlighted access to specimens as a major barrier to research and development, she said, and proposed a mitigation strategy of having regional specimen sharing guided by legal agreements and standards for how high-quality samples are collected, stored, and used.[3] It is also possible for similar agreements to be set up between industry partners and individual countries if concerns of benefit sharing can be worked out among each side. Models of sample sharing agreements are already being developed in the Americas (through the Pan American Health Organization [PAHO]), Europe (through the European Union), and Africa (through the Africa Centres for Disease Con-

---

[3] Standardization considerations that Lackritz shared include specimen characterization and availability for research and development, assessment of diagnostic tests, and evaluation of laboratory proficiency programs; diversity of participant populations (pregnant women, adults, newborns); and specimen type (blood, saliva, urine, amniotic fluid, and cerebrospinal fluid).

trol and Prevention), in conjunction with viral repositories set up during the COVID-19 pandemic), Lackritz noted.One proposed strategy is to have regional specimen sharing guided by legal agreements and standards for how high-quality samples are collected, stored, and used. It is also possible that there may be agreements with industry partners if somehow countries could benefit from providing samples.

Lackritz suggested acting on other elements of a systematic preparedness for the next Zika outbreak, including:

- Developing animal models to recapitulate congenital Zika infection
- Exploring the use of controlled human infection models given the low transmission rate during non-outbreak periods, which would otherwise preclude carrying out necessary research studies
- Preparing geographically and epidemiologically diverse research sites
- Establishing global networks with standardized and pre-approved protocols to be ready for the next outbreak, including working with regulatory and public health agencies in different regions to develop plans for staffing, laboratories, and data management
- Engaging local communities and hearing from women who may participate in trials about how best to implement research in their settings

Conducting longitudinal cohort research would be ideal, said Lackritz, though this research is expensive and difficult to maintain. As a result, Lackritz asserted that strategies for maintaining long-term investment in integrated arbovirus research must be developed. Finally, Lackritz shared that it will be necessary to strengthen epidemiology and surveillance and build global laboratory capacity. Better systems are needed, she continued, for the early detection and monitoring of viral transmission, which in turn can feed into improved models that can be used for forecasting and evaluation. There is also an opportunity to develop a global mapping of reference laboratories, coordination among those laboratories, proficiency testing programs, and standardized protocols to evaluate diagnostics before the next outbreak.

In closing, Lackritz said that reaching these goals will depend on the proper funding. She shared that researchers at the recent international meeting believed it is important to advance Zika research as part of an integrated arbovirus strategy. Other strategies that this group discussed included developing a full public health value proposition with cost–benefit analyses of medical countermeasures and investigating the potential for advanced purchase agreements for vaccines and therapeutics.

OVERVIEW OF ARBOVIRAL DISEASE: THE CURRENT STATUS AND FUTURE OF DISEASE CONTROL

The following session included presentation from four speakers. Marcos Espinal, former assistant director of PAHO, served as moderator and opened the session by commenting that while progress has been made in the control of arboviral diseases, much remains to be done. Duane Gubler, emeritus professor and founding director of the Emerging Infectious Diseases Signature Research Program at Duke-NUS Medical School, Singapore, provided an overview of the global burden of arboviral disease as well as opportunities for advancement in mitigation. The next three speakers focused on specific regions of the world. Laura Kramer, emeritus professor at the University at Albany School of Public Health discussed the threat of endemic and emerging arboviruses in the United States. Sylvain Aldighieri, director of Communicable Diseases Prevention, Control, and Elimination at PAHO, summarized the situation in the Americas, focusing mainly on Latin America. Finally, Raman Velayudhan, head of the Unit on Veterinary Public Health, Vector Control and Environment in the Neglected Tropical Disease Program at the World Health Organization (WHO), spoke about arboviral diseases in the rest of the world with a focus on Africa and Asia.

Gubler began with a comparison of arboviruses with other infectious disease agents. He pointed out that 8 of the 18 high-profile human infectious disease epidemics in the past 30 years were caused by arboviruses, such as dengue, West Nile, Zika, chikungunya, and yellow fever. Furthermore, of the seven pandemics that have occurred in the past 30 years, three have been caused by arboviruses: dengue, chikungunya, and Zika. The take-home message, he said, is that the biggest viral threats in terms of epidemic or pandemic potential are respiratory pathogens, such as SARS-CoV-2, or those spread by urban mosquitoes—that is, arboviruses.

Indeed, he continued, arboviruses are a global threat and not limited to any particular geographic region. Globally, nearly two dozen different types of arbovirus outbreaks were reported in 2023, from dengue, Zika, and chikungunya to Murray Valley encephalitis and Crimean Congo hemorrhagic fever, he said. The three main groups of arboviruses—flaviviruses, alphaviruses, and bunyaviruses—are reflected in these recent outbreaks. He noted that, of the potential diseases caused by pathogens in these groups, those with highest severity and highest probability of occurring are yellow fever, Rift Valley fever, Venezuelan equine encephalitis, Ross River virus infection, and Japanese encephalitis.

Furthermore, Gubler noted that there has been a dramatic increase in epidemic arboviral diseases in the past 30 or 40 years, and attributes this to four major drivers of epidemic transmission. The first driver he cited is demographic changes, particularly population growth and migration patterns. The second is environmental changes, which are closely tied to demographic changes and include unprecedented urban growth, changing lifestyles, and agricultural practices. The third driver is technology, particularly airplanes and shipping containers that have led to the rapid and far-flung movement of people, animals, and pathogens around the world. Finally, the public health infrastructure for handling vector-borne diseases has been allowed to deteriorate globally, he said. Gubler noted that, in combination, these four factors explain much of the increased transmission of arboviral diseases in recent decades.

Gubler highlighted several risk factors for arboviral disease epidemics specifically in urban areas. These include population growth, urbanization, modern modes of transportation, as well as environmental changes such as deforestation, climate, and weather patterns. While he noted that climate and weather are the most important factors in transmission of arboviral diseases, Gubler stressed that unplanned urban growth as a critical risk factor that must be controlled. He elaborated that urban growth and migration have led to the appearance of megacities of 10 to 20 million people, with many of the residents living in slum areas with inadequate housing, water, sewage, other waste management.[4] These crowded conditions provide ideal ecological environments for the maintenance and transmission of viruses and vectors that cause arboviral diseases. These cities also have modern airports through which travelers can access endemic areas where they may be at increased risk of contracting arboviral diseases. Furthermore, Gubler continued, many of these travelers have the potential to introduce exotic viruses into urban areas, potentially amplifying transmission in urban settings."

Gubler went on to share lessons learned from past epidemics. One observation is the cyclic nature of arboviral disease epidemics, and how sometimes long inter-epidemic periods can create a degree of complacency about the diseases, Gubler pointed out. Not only is it easy to forget the diseases when there is no active epidemic and there are no cases being diagnosed, various political and administrative changes can occur during these inter-epidemic periods that result in decreased readiness, such as staff turnover that leads to a loss in expertise and institutional memory. Another lesson, he continued, is that emergency response plans may be ineffective because of inadequate surveillance and because policy makers are often

---

[4] The United Nations defines slum households as dwellings where the inhabitants lack adequate housing or basic services such as access to an improved water source, access to improved sanitation facilities, sufficient living area, housing durability, or security of tenure in the dwelling. See the 2018 UN-Habitat SDG Indicator 11.1.1 Training Module: Adequate Housing and Slum Upgrading. https://unhabitat.org/tools-and-guides (accessed July 11, 2024).

hesitant to decide on implementation until there is an emergency. However, by the time the health emergency situation is certain, it is often too late to mount an effective response. Gubler noted that the general pattern in the current society seems to favor not doing anything until the crisis occurs, leading to outcomes that are far worse than if some preparations had been made.

Gubler noted there are tools to control arboviral diseases—some already available and others being developed—that, if used properly, could reverse the trend of emergent arboviral disease epidemics. However, Gubler believed that it will be necessary to apply these tools to prevention instead of relying on reactive control. Gubler believed that coordinated global funding aimed mainly at helping resource-poor countries develop operational and response plans will be a key factor of success. He went on to list several other requirements to complement the global funding support and disease control tools in reversing the arboviral disease epidemic trend. To ensure sustainability of these efforts, countries around the world will need to commit to the program. For example, he explained, countries in endemic areas will need to invest their own money into the prevention and control of these diseases and not rely on international public health agencies for their public health funding. These public health programs will need to be intersectoral, community partnerships that stay in communication with all segments of the society and not just the medical community. Laboratory-based proactive surveillance and urban renewal will also be important. He added that more research to develop better vaccines, therapeutics, diagnostics, insecticides, and surveillance tools will be critical. This in turn could benefit from the support of the community and of governments to develop and maintain these research programs.

In summary, Gubler said that the risk of epidemic arboviral diseases is now the highest in history. More than 500 viruses are known in animals, many of which have the potential to infect humans and domestic animals to cause major epidemics, and there are certainly many more that have yet to be discovered. More emergent epidemic diseases can be expected in the future, he said, but this trend can be reversed if the available tools are put to work in a synergistic way to prevent and control future outbreaks.

COUNTRY AND REGIONAL EXPERIENCE: IMPACTS AND CHALLENGES OF ARBOVIRAL CONTROL

The remainder of the session was devoted to three presentations about experiences in regional arboviral control in the United States, the rest of the Americas, Asia, and Africa.

United States

Kramer began with an overview of medically important arboviruses that can be considered "established threats" to the United States, noting that some of these are endemic to the United States (including territories). There are three types of equine encephalitis caused by alphaviruses that are endemic in the United States: Western equine encephalitis, Eastern equine encephalitis, and Venezuelan equine encephalitis subtype II, also known as Everglades virus. Human cases are rare for these viruses, although there are regular cases in wildlife and domestic animals. There are several endemic mosquito-borne flaviviruses, including West Nile, St. Louis encephalitis, and dengue. West Nile virus, introduced into the United States in 1999, has since become the leading cause of domestic arboviral disease, Kramer pointed out, with an estimated 7 million infections having taken place in the country. Dengue virus poses a significant threat because it is frequently introduced into the United States, she said, in addition to lower levels of local transmission. Endemic Orthobunyaviruses, which cause neurological disease in humans, include La Crosse virus and Jamestown Canyon virus. Other viruses that are not currently endemic but can be considered as established threats to the United States include yellow fever virus, which caused several outbreaks in the 18th century, chikungunya, Zika, Venezuelan equine encephalitis subtype I-B, and the Mayaro viruses.[5] Kramer also cautioned that there are risks for new arboviral threats to become introduced and established in the United States. There are multiple arboviruses that pose a threat to the United States in the future, such as Rift Valley fever virus, Japanese encephalitis virus, and Murray Valley encephalitis virus. There are also multiple mosquito species that can carry various arboviruses in the United States now, Kramer said. These include *Aedes aegypti, Aedes albopictus, Culex pipiens, Culex quinquefasciatus,* and *Culex lactator.*

Kramer suggested six areas to focus efforts on controlling potential introduction or reemergence of these medically important arboviruses: preparation, surveillance, diagnostics, epidemic countermeasures, research, and social science aspects. Preparation involves defining responsibilities, identifying gaps, organizing laboratory capacities, and localizing resources before the next outbreak occurs. Surveillance enables anticipation of the risk of an arboviral epidemic rather than being limited to responding to the outbreak retroactively. Rapid diagnostics enable tracking of an outbreak as it is progressing, and thus it is also important to train people on how to

---

[5] Kramer elaborated that, since 2014, there have been thousands of cases of chikungunya reported in U.S. travelers returning from affected areas in the Americas and a few cases of local transmission reported. There were large outbreaks of Zika in the United States in 2015 and 2016, but there have been no reports of Zika virus being transmitted by mosquitoes since 2018 in the United States.

perform these diagnostic tests before an outbreak appears. Basic epidemic countermeasures include vector control, personal protection, therapeutics, and vaccines. Intensive vector management programs have been effective in reducing the size of outbreaks, Kramer said, but they are costly and typically initiated only after many cases have already occurred. Personal protective measures can also be effective, but adherence to best practices, such as wearing long pants and using insect repellant, is often very low. Ongoing research can address these shortfalls, she said, by developing innovations in surveillance and epidemic countermeasures (e.g., insect control, diagnostics, and vaccines), while also conducting long-term studies on the epidemiology and ecology and geographic distribution of arboviruses in the world. Finally, she said, it is critical to have effective communication networks and commitment from local communities to partner in arboviral disease control. Kramer also noted that success will depend in part on building coalitions of national and global partners who can work together to identify changes in pathogen distribution and genomics, which can in turn provide early signals to public health officials.

To understand the cyclic nature and be able to predict arbovirus emergence, it is necessary to understand the drivers of disease emergence and establishment, Kramer said. This is a complex process that involves both biotic and abiotic factors. The biotic factors include the interactions among the virus, the vector, and the vertebrate host(s). These are shaped by the abiotic factors including the environment, landscape, ecology, agriculture, urbanization, and weather. Furthermore, climate change can affect the range, intensity, and seasonality of vector-borne diseases.

Kramer used West Nile virus as an example to illustrate the complex biotic factors affecting prediction and control in the United States. There are multiple different vectors, vertebrate hosts, and ecological niches associated with this one pathogen. In the southern region of the continental United States, the vector is *Culex quinquefasciatus*, a container breeding mosquito that feeds on both birds and mammals. In the west, the vector is *Culex tarsalis*, a floodwater breeding mosquito that feeds on mammals and birds. In the eastern region, the vector is *Culex pipiens*, a container breeder that feeds mainly on birds. Additionally, *Culex pipiens* has two forms, *Culex pipiens pipiens* and *Culex pipiens molestus*, that have different over-wintering, feeding, and egg laying patterns. Unsurprisingly, the patterns of West Nile infections vary tremendously between the Midwest, the Southwest, and the Northeast, Kramer said, complicating vector control and disease modeling.

In contrast, dengue and other viruses transmitted by *Aedes aegypti* do not require a zoonotic cycle, she noted. These viruses are rapidly transported to new locations because infected humans, a highly mobile vertebrate host, can directly infect the mosquito vectors *Aedes aegypti* and *Aedes albopictus*. These mosquitoes have significantly expanded their ranges to the north and west because of climate change, further increasing the risk of population exposure to dengue and Zika, Kramer said. These arboviruses carried by *Aedes* mosquitoes are also challenging to diagnose, she continued, because early symptoms of diseases caused by these viruses tend to be similar and serologic assays for these viruses tend to cross-react. Distinguishing between the viruses requires specialized techniques such as plaque reduction neutralization, which is expensive, slow, and requires specific training.

Kramer also brought up tick-borne viruses, cautioning that while they are somewhat neglected in discussions so far, they have been expanding in range. Powassan virus is probably the most important tickborne virus in the United States, she said. It is carried by the *Ixodes scapularis* tick that is found across the eastern half of the United States, and the virus is now found across a significant portion of this range. Although there remains fewer than 50 reported cases each year, the incidence of disease has been increasing over the past couple of decades. Other tickborne viruses of concern in the United States are the Heartland virus and the Bourbon virus, Kramer said. The Heartland virus, first identified in Missouri in 2009, causes severe fever with thrombocytopenia; while rare in the U.S., thousands of clinical cases of this disease have been reported in China. The Bourbon virus, first found in 2014 in a sick patient in Bourbon County, Kansas, remains relatively rare.

In conclusion, Kramer noted that a strong public health infrastructure will be crucial, as will global surveillance with international cooperation and sharing of resources and data. Also, "we need to pay more attention to arboviruses on a global scale and viruses that are not as exotic as the *Aedes*-transmitted viruses," she said. Other needs include early and rapid detection and reporting of human and zoonotic disease outbreaks and effective scientific communication, not just with the public but also among scientists and with funding agencies. She acknowledges the importance of taking a One Health approach in addressing arboviruses.[6] Broad, multidisciplinary, long-term research programs will be vital, as will rapid technology transfer from the bench, Kramer stated.

---

[6] One Health is a collaborative, multilevel, transdisciplinary approach to preventing, detecting, preparing for, and responding to outbreaks of infectious disease that recognizes the health of humans, animals, plants, and the wider environment are closely linked and inter-dependent. See https://www.who.int/publications/m/item/one-health-definitions-and-principles (accessed July 4, 2024).

The Americas

Aldighieri discussed how dengue, chikungunya, Zika, and yellow fever have affected the Americas over the past couple of decades and the efforts that have been taken to control these diseases. These viruses are ubiquitous in the Americas year-round, he said. Dengue has caused epidemics in the Americas since the 1980s, while chikungunya was introduced in 2013, and Zika was first detected in 2015 (Espinal et al., 2019). Yellow fever is present in 13 countries, and there are also several emerging arboviruses in the Americas. Aldighieri highlighted two of these emerging viruses, Oropouche and Mayaro, which he said deserve special attention.

Aldighieri noted that the first line of defense against these arboviruses in the Americas are the virus reference laboratories. There are operational reference laboratories in the different subregions throughout the Americas, and there are several national labs, such as the one in Nicaragua, that have significant capacity for the detection and characterization of arboviruses. There is also a network of these laboratories, the Arbovirus Diagnosis Laboratory Network of the Americas (RELDA), that Aldighieri described as a major asset to arboviral preparedness and response. Nonetheless, Aldighieri believed this laboratory network could be strengthened in a few ways: by developing and standardizing laboratory diagnosis algorithms for arboviruses, improving the distribution of reagents for serological and molecular tests, strengthening the laboratory confirmation and identification of serotypes in the countries of the Americas, and further developing the complementary Genomic Surveillance of Dengue Virus in the Americas network (ViGenDA).

Aldighieri shared some lessons learned about patient care and about vector control. With endemic diseases, while the case burden may consistently increase over time, the proportion of severe cases and case fatality rate can be decreased by improving patient care at the primary health care level. This could be accomplished with updated training of health care workers in the management of severe cases, including training them regarding early predictors of when patients are likely to fare poorly. During epidemics, he said, it is key to be able to reorganize health care services and focus more on appropriate triage and preventing deaths. In recent years, investment has been made in virtual training for dengue and chikungunya management, but there is still room for improvement and reducing deaths related to inadequate clinical management.

Regarding vector control, he said, while *Aedes aegypti* has spread to colonize most of the intertropical areas of the Americas after the eradication program failed in the early 1970s, modernizing entomological surveillance methods and improving information systems could still make a major difference in country vector control efforts. In particular, he said it would be valuable to implement integrated vector management, rationally incorporate new technologies and approaches, and strengthen capacities for monitoring and managing insecticide resistance. One challenge in vector control is the population growth and increase in the number of large cities that has taken place over the past several decades. Inhabitants in the Latin America and the Caribbean region increased from 168 million inhabitants in 1950 to over 660 million in 2022, and currently 80 percent of these people live in large cities (ECLAC, 2022). During the Zika response in 2016, Aldighieri said, "We estimated that more than 500 million people were at risk to be infected by the virus through *Aedes aegypti*." In addition, climate change is leading to an expansion of the geographic areas with conditions suitable for vector reproduction.

Elaborating on the effects of climate change on the suitability of environments for disease vectors, Aldighieri cited the results of a recent study that found the world became more suitable for the development of *Aedes aegypti* at a rate of 1.5 percent per decade between 1950 and 2000, a trend that is expected to increase to 3.2–4.4 percent per decade by 2050 (Iwamura et al., 2020). As a result, the expansion of the vector into North America is expected to accelerate to around 2–6 kilometers per year by 2050. He noted an equity concern in this future scenario, stressing the unequal impacts of arboviral diseases across different groups. For example, Aldighieri noted that the incidence rates of dengue are, on average, much higher in people with low literacy levels than in people with high literacy levels. Similarly, Aldighieri explained that dengue rates are far higher among people with less access to basic health services.

To address this growing threat, Aldighieri described an integrated management strategy for the prevention and control of arboviral diseases that PAHO has been implementing on behalf of its member states for almost 20 years. This strategy was initiated to deal with dengue and later expanded to address chikungunya and Zika. The strategy draws from lessons of past arboviral epidemics, though Aldighieri noted that the strategy may need to be reassessed considering the recent changes in the region, including population growth and climate change.

To illustrate some of the concerns about the spread of arboviruses and strategies that could be used to resist that spread, Aldighieri described the reemergence of yellow fever in 2016–2017 in southeast Brazil that has led to more than 3,500 laboratory-confirmed cases and more than 900 deaths. The best way to predict where a yellow fever outbreak will occur, Aldighieri said, is to monitor for yellow fever epizootic episodes, or outbreaks among animal populations, and use information on those epizootic episodes to guide vaccination campaigns. Public health officials in southeast and south Brazil were able to dramatically reduce the number of human cases of yellow fever with this approach. Aldighieri detailed additional reasons behind this successful outcome. In particular, this outbreak was transmitted by sylvatic vectors (i.e., via nonhuman primates and non-*Aedes* mosquitoes) and did not involve the *Aedes aegypti* vector in an urban setting. The context of the outbreak was deforestation and canopy loss, and much of the disease transmission took place along sylvatic corridors that sometimes run very close to urban areas, where epizootic spread can take place at a high velocity. Aldighieri also noted that it is best to take a One Health approach to addressing this type of outbreak, where it is critical to consider the integrated health of people, animals, and ecosystems. Given the important roles that deforestation, sylvatic corridors, and nonhuman primates play in the spread of the yellow fever virus and its ultimate threat to humans, the traditional approach of focusing narrowly on mosquitoes and human patients is not the best way to control and respond to outbreaks.

In his conclusion, Aldighieri emphasized several takeaway messages: The region of the Americas encompasses a constant circulation of emerging and reemerging arboviruses, many with high epidemic potential, and this presents a permanent risk to public health. Second, while the case number of diseases like dengue have consistently increased, countries have been able to reduce the proportion of cases that progress to severe disease and reduce the number of deaths from the disease through systematic capacity-building efforts. Finally, laboratory networks must be strengthened and used to detect the emergence of new viruses as well as monitoring existing viruses.

Worldwide

Almost 4 billion people in nearly 130 countries around the world are at risk of *Aedes*-borne arboviral infections, Velayudhan said, and the public health threat posed by these diseases is growing. For instance, the worldwide incidence of dengue increased tenfold over the past two decades, reaching a record high of 5.2 million cases reported in 129 countries in 2019 (WHO, 2023). Dengue outbreaks continued to be reported in many countries during the COVID-19 pandemic, leading WHO to create the Global Arbovirus Initiative. Metrics for 2023 have also been alarming, Velayudhan said, with reports of more than 5 million cases of dengue across 80 countries and in all WHO regions. While the overall case fatality rate is low, with at least 5,000 dengue-related deaths estimated for the year (WHO, 2023), Velayudhan reiterated that "any death is a matter of grave concern." As of December 2023, WHO is actively monitoring dengue outbreaks in 23 countries, 17 of which are in the Americas.

Turning to Southeast Asia, he said, 10 out of the 11 countries in this region are dengue endemic. Recently there has been a significant increase in cases in Bangladesh, from a little over 62,000 in 2022 to over 310,000 in 2023, while the number of deaths there surpassed 1,600. Thailand also had an unusually high number of cases—over 135,000—in 2023. Case fatality rates ranged from 0.04 percent in Nepal to 0.72 in Indonesia. Most of the data in this region come from hospitalized or severe cases. In the western Pacific regions, 2023 was a bad year as well. Eight countries in the region reported dengue cases, with the Philippines and Vietnam having particularly high numbers (WHO, 2024).

There are relatively little data for the eastern Mediterranean region, but there is growing interest in stepping up surveillance in the region, Velayudhan said. In 2023, eight countries reported a total of 10 dengue outbreaks in the Mediterranean region. It is a challenging area because of ongoing armed hostilities, which limit the amount and timeliness of information on infections, but the available data indicate a systematic increase in the number of cases. There has been an upsurge of dengue infections in Saudi Arabia, while Djibouti, Somalia, and Sudan have experienced outbreaks for the past several years. Afghanistan recorded its first outbreak in 2019. In Europe, dengue is not endemic and the recorded cases are mostly travel-related. Still, dengue has been reported constantly since 2000, and in 2011 there was a major outbreak on Madeira Island. In 2023 there were 81 cases in Italy, 43 in France, and 3 in Spain, which Velayudhan characterized as a "matter of concern" because it is very unusual to have three different countries report cases in the same year. Furthermore, there was local transmission in those countries. The mosquitoes that carry the virus hibernate in the winter, but the next summer's potential for outbreaks is significant, Velayudhan said.

The African region is among the top four regions most affected by dengue and in 2020 recorded more than 200,000 cases, but it is not possible at this time to know the exact burden there. Some 30 countries in the region are dengue prone, and since the beginning of 2023, 11 countries in Africa have reported outbreaks of the disease. One of the countries of greatest concern is Burkina Faso, which had over 170,000 suspected cases of dengue, and 760 deaths (WHO, 2022). Velayudhan noted that the region is working to establish a surveillance system for arboviruses, and in 2022 a regional framework for combatting arboviruses and other vector-borne diseases was approved.

Velayudhan attributed the upsurge in dengue and other arboviruses in these regions to a combination of factors. Greater mobility and increased travel make it easier for the viruses to move from one area to another and increase the chances of outbreaks. The El Niño phenomenon brings higher temperatures, higher humidity, and greater rainfall to many areas, making the environments more suitable for mosquitoes. Environmental factors, such as urbanization, population growth, and the mass migration of populations also play a role, while complex humanitarian crises and armed conflicts weaken health systems and make access to health care facilities more difficult. The co-circulation of the four serotypes of dengue may lead to an increased number of severe dengue cases and deaths because of the effects of antibody-dependent enhancement following secondary infection.[7]

Those who seek to monitor and control dengue and other arboviruses face many challenges, Velayudhan said. The biggest is insufficient multisectoral coordination for dengue responses at national and local levels. "Within a country it is becoming increasingly challenging to work across ministries and to implement the program and monitor it for a particular period," he said. A second challenge is that there are relatively few effective tools for dealing with dengue. There are no sustainable vector control tools, vaccines have limited effectiveness, and there are no drugs to treat or prevent disease. The presence of multiple outbreaks—COVID-19, global cholera, and others—combined with other humanitarian crises all taking place simultaneously has greatly stretched resources, both financial and workforce. This is exacerbated by capacity issues, particularly a lack of trained clinical, entomological, and vector control staff.

Clinical diagnosis remains a priority issue, he continued, because most of the cases are asymptomatic. At the same time there is inadequate management of cases, and the triaging of cases is a particular challenge in many countries. A related issue is the limited capacities for laboratory testing, though Velayudhan noticed that COVID-19 seems to have spurred the development of new and easier-to-perform diagnostics, especially multiplex assays, so this may become less of a problem. Making further progress against arboviral diseases around the world will require thinking outside of the box, he continued. For instance, producers of water storage containers should be encouraged to develop ways to ensure that a lid is always covering the container except when it is in use. Along those lines, WHO is working with the United Nations to make sure that all refugee camps have their tanks well covered.

Looking to the future, Velayudhan anticipated that many cities will likely experience water stress and even water depletion, and this is likely to trigger more dengue as people hoard water in and around their houses. Building on experiences from the past, he added, during outbreaks public health authorities should make a concerted effort to address the periphery first, keeping mosquito populations low in the areas adjoining the hotspots as a way of preventing spread of the virus. Risk communication and community engagement efforts should focus on conveying a single important message, reinforcing it year after year, and the communication should be

---

[7] For an explanation on the phenomenon of antibody-dependent enhancement in dengue infections, see https://www.nature.com/scitable/topicpage/host-response-to-the-dengue-virus-22402106/ (accessed July 4, 2024).

done in the local language. Targeted interventions are needed to protect the most vulnerable populations.

In conclusion, Velayudhan offered several take-home messages:

- Vectors are continuing to expand into new countries.
- Enhancing real-time integrated surveillance will be essential to preventing outbreaks.
- Prevention should be prioritized, including vector population reduction wherever possible.
- Programmatic approaches can be more sustainable than outbreak response.

In particular, Velayudhan commented that a programmatic approach is needed for dengue because it is no longer an outbreak disease; it is endemic in more than 100 countries. Urban environments are hot spots for the rapid spread of diseases, and urbanization is only going to increase in the future, especially in continental Africa. Thus, a greater focus on urban environment and urban health could be beneficial. Finally, he said, tailored interventions along with infrastructure and capacity building will be essential in the effective control of arboviral diseases.

DISCUSSION

In the discussion session, one participant referred to the importance of taking a One Health approach to control arboviral diseases and asked the panelists to discuss how they would operationalize One Health in this context. Kramer stated that to control the spread of West Nile virus and other related viruses, it is important to study the virus, birds, mosquitoes, and human behavior. "We need to understand the migration patterns of the birds, the seasonality of them, the feeding patterns of mosquitoes on the birds, and of course the vector capacity of the birds, how infectious are they for how long." For mosquitoes, she continued, one must think about how to control all the stages of the mosquito—the larva, the eggs, and the adults. Aldighieri added that it is also crucial to consider environmental factors, including wildlife. Surveillance systems used for different purposes must be harmonized, he said. Surveillance in farming systems, for instance, has different interests than surveillance for human public health. However, some new tools, such as genomic surveillance, can create a bridge between the different systems, Aldighieri said. There is a policy framework developed in the Americas for bridging the different sectors necessary for the One Health Approach, led by a permanent forum called RMSA after the Spanish acronym for the Conference of the Ministries of Health and Ministries of Agriculture of the Americas. It provides a place for various stakeholders and decision makers to share opinions and make decisions. Gubler thought that One Health is a "buzz word" that is used liberally in scholarly publications as a solution without providing additional details; however, he recognized parallels between the One Health approach and the study of disease ecology, where disease transmission cycles, ecology, animal life cycles, and human-animal interactions are examined collectively.

Panelists were also asked about how they would prioritize making investments in the various unmet needs that had been mentioned, such as diagnostic capacity, surveillance systems, communication, and research and development. Kramer answered that those things are all high priority. However, she emphasized the importance of early-warning surveillance systems in moving from a reactive to a proactive approach. "With a zoonotic virus, once the virus is in the wildlife," she said, "there's no way of really controlling it, which we saw with West Nile." Unfortunately, she continued, the current surveillance system is very inefficient and expensive. Additionally, Gubler noted that it would be useful to pay attention to surveillance and epidemiology news from other countries as part of understanding or predicting the threat that those outbreaks might pose in the United States.

Gubler agreed that preparation is a critical area where investment is needed and noted that existing early warning systems are not very effective. He focused on prevention, which requires applying principles of disease ecology to determine the best leverage points to intervene in the transmission cycle to prevent or reduce transmission. Since there is probably no single preventive approach that will fit all scenarios, he believed the best method will be to "develop an integrated approach with synergistic interventions that work to reduce transmission." Gubler stated that to do that will require coming back to the One Health or disease ecology approaches to understand the complex interactions that go into epidemic transmission.

REFERENCES

CDC (Centers for Disease Control and Prevention). 2024. Transmission of Zika virus. https://www.cdc.gov/zika/php/transmission/index.html (accessed October 15, 2024).

ECLAC (Economic Commission for Latin America and the Caribbean). 2022. *Demographic Observatory of Latin America and the Caribbean 2022. Population Trends in Latin America and the Caribbean: Demographic Effects of the Covid-19 Pandemic.* (LC/PUB.2022/13-P) Santiago: United Nations.

Espinal, M. A., J. K. Andrus, B. Jauregui, S. H. Waterman, D. M. Morens, J. I. Santos, O. Horstick, L. A. Francis, and D. Olson. 2019. Emerging and reemerging *Aedes*-transmitted arbovirus infections in the region of the Americas: Implications for health policy. *American Journal of Public Health* 109(3):387–392. https://doi.org/10.2105/ajph.2018.304849.

Iwamura, T., A. Guzman-Holst, and K. A. Murray. 2020. Accelerating invasion potential of disease vector *Aedes aegypti* under climate change. *Nature Communications* 11(1):2130.

WHO (World Health Organization). 2022. *Framework for the Integrated Control, Elimination and Eradication of Tropical and Vector-Borne Diseases in the African Region 2022-2030*. Lomé, Togo: World Health Organization.

WHO. 2023. *Dengue—global situation*. https://www.who.int/emergencies/disease-outbreak-news/item/2023-DON498 (accessed July 11, 2024).

WHO. 2024. *Global dengue surveillance*. https://worldhealthorg.shinyapps.io/dengue_global/ (accessed July 11, 2024).

3

Assessing and Detecting Arboviral Risk

Highlights

- The World Health Organization (WHO) is working to develop an integrated global arbovirus reporting system that will collect, aggregate, and analyze data from around the world. (Rojas)
- There are large gaps between different regions in their capabilities to collect, analyze, and report data and to act on those data. Improving the global surveillance system will require helping the countries that are lagging improve the capabilities. (Rojas)
- There has been exponential growth in the amount of genomic data on arboviruses published over the past three decades. These data enable genomic epidemiology. (Faria)
- Genomic data can be used in near-real time to analyze the dynamics of an outbreak. Such data can also improve forecasting. (Faria)
- Singapore uses a multiprong approach to control dengue, with two aimed at keeping the mosquito population low and the other two intended to break the transmission chain once cases of dengue have appeared. (Ng)
- Knowing the genotypes of the prevalent viruses can provide important information both for tracking and implementing control efforts. (Ng)

continued

- Models can be valuable in predicting the likely spread of a virus and in proving the value of surveillance and control efforts. (Ng)
- Diagnostic testing can play a major role in arbovirus mitigation, and, indeed, dengue diagnostics are now on the WHO essential diagnostics list. (Boeras)
- Multiplex diagnostic tests that look for multiple arboviruses have promise for both patient management and surveillance. (Boeras)

NOTE: These points were made by the individual workshop speakers/participants identified above. They are not intended to reflect a consensus among workshop participants.

Eva Harris, professor of infectious diseases and vaccinology at the University of California, Berkeley, chaired the second session on current and forward-thinking strategies of assessing and detecting arboviral risk, specifically through surveillance and diagnostics. "I think we're at a really exciting place," she said, because of the variety of techniques, particularly molecular and genomics methods, for tracking and diagnosing arboviruses and arboviral diseases.

The panel consisted of four presenters. Diana Rojas, technical officer in the Epidemic and Pandemic Preparedness and Prevention Department at the World Health Organization (WHO), spoke on epidemiological surveillance. Nuno Faria, professor of viral genomic epidemiology in the School of Public Health at Imperial College London, discussed genomic surveillance. Lee Ching Ng, group director of the Environmental Health Institute at Singapore's National Environment Agency, spoke about integrated surveillance and risk assessment in Singapore. Finally, Rosanna Peeling, professor emeritus at the London School of Hygiene and Tropical Medicine and the founding director of the International Diagnostic Center Network, was scheduled to speak but could not attend, so her presentation—with additional contributions—was made by Debi Boeras, founder and chief executive officer of the Global Health Impact Group. She spoke about the role that diagnostics can play in arbovirus surveillance and mitigation.

EPIDEMIOLOGICAL SURVEILLANCE

Rojas began by describing WHO's Global Arbovirus Initiative, a six-pillar plan to tackle mosquito-borne viruses with epidemic and pandemic potential in an integrated way. The first pillar, monitoring and anticipating risk, would be the subject of her talk, and she quickly described the other five pillars before returning to the first. The second pillar is reducing epidemic risk at the local level through actions such as strengthening early-detection capacities at the local level, this would include not just improved lab detection but also improving the abilities of health care workers to identify these diseases early in their course. The third pillar is strengthening vector control, including improvements in environmental surveillance. The fourth is preventing and preparing for pandemics, particularly through global coordination and data sharing as well as building more prepared and resilient populations. Fifth is enhancing innovation and new approaches; this refers mainly to strengthening research on vaccines, therapeutics, new vector control tools, and the transmission dynamics of arboviruses. Sixth is building a coalition of partners. "If we all have the same goal, if we all have the same priorities, we will be more likely to succeed," Rojas said.

Turning her attention back to the first pillar—monitoring risk and anticipation—Rojas said that the pillar has two priority actions associated with it. The first is to develop a global risk monitoring framework for arboviruses using a One Health approach, and the second is to use that framework to forecast and model potential epidemic and pandemic scenarios for arboviruses. WHO has been working on a data dashboard as part of this first pillar. WHO first developed an inventory of the data services and systems across the WHO regions and is now working on an integrated arbovirus reporting system that would capture arbovirus-related data from the local level, aggregate them, and send them to the regional level and ultimately to the global level. With those data, the next step would be to then design and operationalize a global arbovirus dashboard that would be hosted by WHO headquarters. However, Rojas said, there are some regions that are more advanced in arbovirus surveillance architecture than others. Due to delays and additional complexities from the COVID-19 pandemic, WHO worked with the London School of Hygiene and Tropical Medicine to develop two tools in parallel. The first was to build a data dashboard with individual regions, and the second was to create an integrated risk map with a model including environmental data and other open data sources that can give a quick risk assessment of the situation. Rojas demonstrated a draft of the integrated risk map.[1] "We are trying to do a hotspot mapping for all the zoonotic and epidemic pathogens with epidemic and pandemic potential," she explained, which included avian influenza, SARS, and Rift Valley fever. The next step will be to validate these hotspot maps.

In its work with the individual regions on data dashboards, WHO has realized different capacities at the different regions. The Pan American

---

[1] https://experience.arcgis.com/experience/31ff667796be41f8b4e2cd0393e44bfe/ (accessed February 4, 2024).

Health Organization (PAHO) has one of the most complete surveillance systems on arboviruses, Rojas said, including open data that allow real-time monitoring of this information through PLISA, the Spanish acronym for the Health Information Platform for the Americas. PAHO has been sharing their experience with other regions, and now the southeast Asia region is publishing a bulletin and working on its dashboard, as is the western Pacific region.

In 2021, WHO carried out a global capacity survey for the surveillance, prevention, and control of arboviral diseases, and 167 countries and territories participated. The survey found major inequalities both within and between countries. "We have countries that moved completely from paper-based to computer-based surveillance or even real-time surveillance using cell phones, iPads, and computers," Rojas said. "But then you have some that are still using paper," and transferring the information on paper to digital format can pose a significant challenge to effective surveillance.

Similarly, while some countries report their data in real or near-real time, others report quarterly or even yearly. While this can be sufficient for program evaluation, it is not adequate for monitoring outbreaks or pathogens with epidemic or pandemic potential, Rojas noted. Thus, WHO is working with several countries to help them gather and report their data in a timelier fashion. Another issue is that while some countries are able to collect the data, they do not have the personnel or the tools to conduct analysis of these data. WHO is also working to bring analytic tools to the local level so that health authorities can take advantage of the data they have gathered. Data analysis is basic to informing early warning systems, Rojas noted. A separate issue is that some countries have early warning systems but ministries of health are not using the data. The question, then, is how to get countries to take action based on the surveillance outcomes. Another problem in some countries, she added, is that epidemiological surveillance is isolated from other surveillance systems. In those cases, it is important to integrate the epidemiological surveillance data with laboratory surveillance data, including data from genomic surveillance, entomological surveillance, and environmental surveillance. Finally, in some countries there is little or no action taken even when an alert is triggered by arboviral disease surveillance.

Rojas noted some gaps and opportunities in improving surveillance on a regional level. In some regions, for instance, there are no regional agreements on arbovirus surveillance. In those cases, the countries should agree on standard case definitions, which basic variables should be shared, what confirmatory tests should be given, and how information is shared. One challenge is that some countries are worried that reporting on arboviruses will affect tourism. There should be people in each region who are working to drive arbovirus surveillance processes.

On the global level, Rojas said that there are also several steps that can be taken to improve surveillance globally. "We need to fill the gaps and inequities in technology across the globe to guarantee timely or real-time surveillance," she said, and analytical tools need to be transferred to the local levels to improve response. Such tools could include early-warning systems, modeling, and genomic surveillance, among others. Lessons learned from the capacities built during the COVID-19 response should be used in improving surveillance capabilities for other diseases, such as arboviral diseases. Using an integrated approach like One Health to monitor and control arboviral diseases will be crucial, as will taking a multisectoral approach at all levels. Other factors in strengthening the control of and response to arboviral diseases are increasing awareness of those diseases, building trust with communities, and maintaining continuous financial support. Finally, Rojas said, laboratories and surveillance systems must be prepared now before outbreaks emerge.

GENOMIC SURVEILLANCE

Faria gave an overview of current efforts in genomic surveillance, beginning with details on the degree of genomic surveillance conducted for different arboviruses. The more viral genomes known, the more details one can infer about the spread of that virus. In the case of dengue, about 3,000 genomes were sequenced in 2023 alone, Faria said, which corresponds to about seven genomes per million dengue cases. Compared to other pathogens, the number of genomes sequenced for dengue is relatively high, and this is certainly higher than the number of genomes sequenced for other arboviruses such as West Nile and chikungunya viruses. Faria noted that Zika is among the least sequenced arbovirus among these pathogens of concern.

Over the past several decades, there has been exponential growth in the number of genome sequences submitted for arboviral pathogens (Figure 3-1). The first arboviral sequence shared in the National Center for Biotechnology Information's GeneBank was for yellow fever in 1986. Venezuelan equine encephalitis, West Nile, and dengue genomes followed in 1993, then chikungunya in 1994, and Zika in 2005. More than 20,000 arboviral genomes have been reported up to this point—for dengue, West Nile, chikungunya, Zika, yellow fever, and Venezuelan equine encephalitis, Faria said. If the exponential increase were to continue, he anticipates there would be 250,000 arboviral genomes available within 10 years (Sayer et al., 2023).

The source of viral genome data is also not equally distributed between the pathogens and endemic countries. Brazil produces more sequences for chikungunya, yellow fever, and Zika than any other country, while

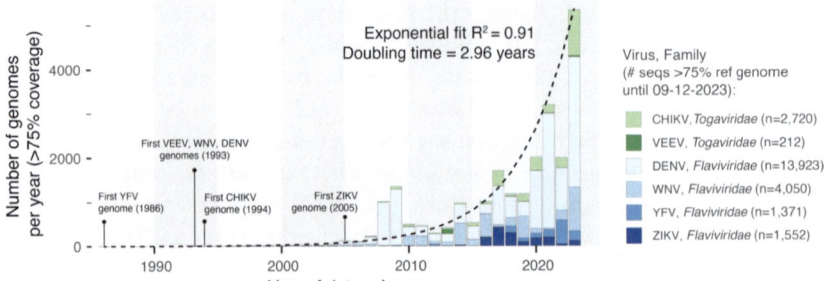

FIGURE 3-1 Exponential growth of genomic sequencing data for arboviral threats.
NOTES: CHIKV = chikungunya virus; DENV = dengue virus; VEEV = Venezuelan equine encephalitis virus; WNV = west Nile virus; YFV = yellow fever virus; ZIKV = Zika virus.
SOURCES: Presented by Nuno Faria on December 12, 2023; generated from data in NCBI GenBank and Sayers et al., 2023 by Prof. Nuno R. Faria and Dr. Charles Whittaker.

Thailand leads in the number of dengue sequences produced. Indeed, 82 percent of all dengue sequences published online were produced by just 10 countries—Thailand, Vietnam, China, Brazil, Singapore, Nicaragua, Cambodia, the United States, Venezuela, and India. It is difficult to know exactly how representative the resulting arboviral dataset is relative to the underlying burden of disease and the actual number of cases for these different arboviruses, Faria said.[2] However, it is possible to compare estimates of force of infection—the rate at which susceptible individuals in a population acquire an infection—against the number of sequenced genomes per capita in a population. This makes it possible to identify which countries have a high force of infection, but a low number of viral genomes sequenced to determine where to target investments in sequencing. Faria shared that this analysis has identified the Philippines, Jamaica, and El Salvador as countries where it would be beneficial to do more genomic sequencing of dengue and other arboviruses.

Faria went on to describe that there are two main strategies in genomic sequencing to maximize the public health benefit: untargeted sequencing and targeted sequencing. Untargeted sequencing, also known as metagenomics or pathogen-agnostic surveillance, does not require a prior knowl-

---

[2] Faria also discussed that disease transmission dynamics of different virus influence the ease of detection and, relatedly, the quantity of genomes sequenced. Of note, Zika viral titers in human samples are on average significantly lower compared with titers of chikungunya, dengue, or yellow fever viruses. Faria pointed to this as part of the reason for why there are so few Zika genomes available.

edge of the pathogen genome to be investigated, he said. Instead, with this approach all the genetic material found within a sample is sequenced and assembled into full or partial genomes for analysis. Targeted sequencing, on the other hand, needs a priori knowledge of the viral genome that is being sought. For example, Faria said, untargeted sequencing was used to generate the first genomes of SARS-CoV-2 in Wuhan, China, and it is very useful for identifying (potentially unknown) pathogens in the early stage of an outbreak. Targeted sequencing is typically used at a later stage of an outbreak or an epidemic and can help provide epidemiological understanding of viral lineages.

Knowledge of the genome sequence of a virus unlocks many applications, Faria said. It can help in designing diagnostics, therapeutics, and vaccines, and it is useful for investigating phenotypic changes, such as a mutation in the chikungunya that increases its transmissibility in *Aedes albopictus*. For arboviruses, he said, genome sequences could be valuable for investigating their drivers of emergence, persistence, and evolution. One key application is genomic epidemiology that leverages these sequence data to study the distribution and spread of pathogens. There are four key components of genomic epidemiology, Faria said. It starts with sequencing viral genomes from samples that were identified as positive for the presence of the pathogen by polymerase chain reaction (PCR) and have appropriate metadata. The next step is bioinformatics, which typically involves phylogenetic inference using both outbreak and background sequences. In many cases, this is a major bottleneck in the overall process. Next are genetic analyses, where researchers investigate how transmission likely took place over time and reconstruct the evolutionary history of a given pathogen. It is normally done using samples recovered from human patients, but in the case of zoonotic or epizootic cycles the viruses may have come from mosquitoes, nonhuman primates, or other sources. The fourth step is translation into public health action. There are many open questions on how to best approach this, Faria said, but dashboards and visualizations have proved helpful in things like investigating transmissibility and the severity of viral lineages and making forecasts.

To illustrate ways that genomic information can be used in arbovirus surveillance, Faria shared an example from 2016 where detection of Zika virus and its potential origin was optimized using climate-informed temporal sampling. There were many samples available for testing with very limited time, so his group used a map of suitability for *Aedes* mosquitoes to determine which samples they would test (Faria et al., 2017). That process allowed them to recover about 54 genomes for Zika during a 2-week period. By comparing these 54 genomes with another 200 Zika genomes, they discovered that Zika had been introduced into Brazil from French Polynesia in a single event and, more importantly, that it had been circulating undetected for over 1 year across Brazil and across other countries before it was first detected in May 2015.

In another study, Faria's group collaborated with the Angolan Ministry of Health to sequence Zika samples and showed that the virus strains circulating in Angola were connected to strains circulating in northeast Brazil. Then, using mobility data such as the number of monthly air passengers to Angola, they showed that air travel was linked to the spread of the Zika virus and, specifically, that the Asian lineage of the Zika virus was linked to continental Africa and Angola (Hill et al., 2019). Another team sequenced 39 Zika genomes from a 2016 outbreak in Florida, identified four lineages, and determined an R_0 of between 0.5 and 0.8 that allowed them to estimate a very low probability that Zika would persist for over 1 year in Florida.[3] Furthermore, they were also able to hypothesize that there were about 40 separate introductions of the Zika virus in Miami alone (Grubaugh et al., 2017). The value of genomics data is illustrated in another study, still in preparation in late 2023, where he and colleagues compared the performance of different forecast models for dengue outbreaks with and without genomic information on the various strains. What they have found, he said, is that all forecasts seem to improve when they consider phylogenetic data in the model.

Faria discussed the yellow fever outbreak in 2017 in Brazil as an exemplar of the importance of using genomic surveillance in understanding the source of arbovirus outbreaks.[4] It was the largest outbreak in Brazil in the past 8 years, Faria said, and within 5 days he and his team analyzed 50–60 sequences from nonhuman primates and from humans to investigate whether the outbreak was due to an urban transmission cycle or sylvatic transmission (Faria et al., 2018). "Essentially what we saw using phylogenetic approaches, within 5 days upon arrival," he said, "was that every human sequence was clustering very closely to a nonhuman primate sequence, indicating frequent cross-species transmission from nonhuman primates to humans" in a sylvatic transmission via non-*Aedes* mosquitoes. Faria also described an example of work done with untargeted sequencing. When a colony of 68 Alouatta monkeys in a São Paulo Park died within a short period in 2017–2018, Faria and team used untargeted sequencing to simultaneously identify the yellow fever virus that was responsible for their deaths and the mosquito species that had infected them with the virus.

In closing, Faria pointed to areas that need work in the future. There is potential for greater optimization of global detection or arboviral threats,

---

[3] R_0 is a measure of inherent transmissibility of a pathogen in a fully susceptible population, estimating the number of people that one infected person will transmit the disease to. See https://globalhealth.harvard.edu/understanding-predictions-what-is-r-naught/ (accessed July 11, 2024).

[4] This outbreak was also referenced by Aldighieri in Chapter 2 as an example of taking a One Health approach in outbreak response.

he said, that could involve considering climate, mobility, force of infection, serological estimates, and sampling strategies as well as focusing on under-sampled locations with high transmission rates. There is also potential for models to integrate genomic data with other surveillance data (epidemiological, serological, mobility, entomological, and climate) to improve forecasts for arboviral disease outbreaks. Faria addressed the role of genomics data in developing future low-cost, temperature-insensitive diagnostic tools to improve arboviral surveillance. He concluded by noting the importance of collaborative surveillance across sectors, emergency cycles, and different geographic levels.

INTEGRATED SURVEILLANCE AND RISK ASSESSMENT: CASE STUDY FROM SINGAPORE

Lee Ching Ng began her description of integrated surveillance and risk assessment of dengue in Singapore by providing some background and context: The three crucial elements in the spread of dengue are the virus itself, mosquitoes, and people. Removing any one of the three will stop the spread of the dengue. At this point in time, the only way to control dengue is to control its spread by mosquitoes. Ng noted the importance of clarity in how the three critical elements of an outbreak interact and affect one another in order to understand the epidemic potential of the virus. The latter is particularly challenging, she said, and involves such things as understanding the immunity of the population, the epidemiology of the disease, and various environmental risk factors such as rainfall and temperature.

A typical outbreak begins with a single case, which then spreads to others to form a cluster, which, if it is not controlled, leads to an outbreak. Efforts to prevent outbreaks can take place on many different levels, Ng said. Accurately diagnosing a patient who has dengue and notifying the appropriate authorities can help prevent an individual case from leading to a cluster, for instance, and prompt intervention to minimize further transmission can prevent a cluster from leading to an outbreak. Singapore's dengue control framework has four pillars: surveillance, prevention and control, outbreak management, and public communications and advocacy. The first two are aimed at keeping the mosquito population low, while the second two are intended to break the transmission chain once cases of dengue have appeared (Aik et al., 2019; Ho et al., 2023; Sim et al., 2020). Ng focused on Singapore's surveillance efforts in the remainder of her presentation.

One aspect of Singapore's dengue surveillance is mandatory reporting of positive results from clinicians and laboratories. Since 2008, when the rapid diagnostic test for dengue (based on the non-structural protein antigen 1, or NS1) became available, the health authorities in Singapore have been strongly encouraging doctors to use it on patients who present with the appropriate symptoms, and its increasing use has allowed health officials to get a clearer picture of where dengue is appearing. When a patient tests positive with the NS1 antigen test (run using patient blood samples), the laboratory proceeds to determine the virus's serotype and sequence its genome. In the case of a negative result, the patient sample is subjected to PCR tests for other flaviviruses and chikungunya; many cases of Zika and chikungunya have been discovered this way, Ng added.

The data on dengue infections collected through the NS1 tests are used for public alerts. The public health department maps locations of the cases with a geographic information system (GIS); then, if two cases are discovered within 150 meters of each other within 2 weeks, it is considered to be a cluster, and the existence of a cluster and its location is made available on the National Environment Agency's website.[5] A user can input an address or postal code on the website and see an alert if there is an cluster in that area. People can use this information and implement precautionary measures, such as using insect repellant or wearing long sleeves, she said. Those people who may not use the website are alerted through banners placed around the city. A red banner indicates that there are more than 10 cases in the surrounding area, so care should be taken to avoid infection. A yellow banner indicates fewer than 10 cases in the area, while green indicates that the threat is minimal.

The information obtained from dengue virus serotyping has also proven useful, Ng said. Testing has shown that Singapore has all four serotypes of the virus circulating and that the relative prevalence of the four types provides important information. When the predominant serotype switches from one to another, it is a signal that an outbreak may occur in about 3 months (Rajarethinam et al., 2018). Finally, knowing the genotypes of the prevalent viruses can provide important information. Ng pointed to an outbreak of chikungunya in Singapore in 2008 which had a mutation that allowed the virus to adapt to *Aedes albopictus* as well as *Aedes aegypti* (Ng et al., 2009). Since *Aedes albopictus* is typically encountered outside, in contrast with *Aedes aegypti* that is mostly encountered inside, the public health department had to modify its control measures to focus more on outdoor efforts.

In recent years, Ng said, Singapore has complemented its clinical surveillance with wastewater surveillance that was set up during the COVID-19 pandemic to track the levels of the SARS-CoV-2 virus. Since Zika virus is shed in urine, the National Environment Agency decided to see whether it was also possible for wastewater surveillance to detect the presence of

---

[5] https://www.nea.gov.sg/dengue-zika/dengue/dengue-clusters (accessed July 11, 2024).

Zika. When a small cluster of about 20 Zika cases appeared, the agency found that the data from wastewater did track well with the cases and with the presence of Zika in mosquito surveillance. Conversely, there was no evidence of Zika transmission in people where the wastewater surveillance for Zika was negative. Thus, Ng stated that the wastewater testing offers a reliable way of monitoring for Zika and aids in targeting vector control efforts. Unfortunately, infected patients do not have high shedding of dengue virus in bodily fluids, and wastewater testing for dengue have not proven effective.

As part of their surveillance efforts, Singapore health authorities also test mosquitoes for dengue. Traditionally they have tested mosquito larva, sending out health officers to homes to find larvae and bring them back for testing, but since 2017–2018 they have used a Gravitrap surveillance system (Ong et al., 2021). The Gravitrap has a sticky lining that immobilizes mosquitoes that are then removed by health officers for laboratory testing. There are currently 70,000 such traps distributed around Singapore's 700 square kilometers. Since 90 percent of the residents live in high-rise apartments, traps are placed on lower floors, middle floors, and upper floors in order to get a full understanding of the distribution of the mosquitoes. It traps both *Aedes aegypti*, the usual carrier of dengue, and *Aedes albopictus*, a recently emerged vector for dengue. Analyses done on these data indicate the threshold for dengue transmission is about five infected *Aedes aegypti* mosquitoes caught per 100 traps. When the number does go above a high-risk threshold, the department posts warnings on its website and with banners around the area to caution the public of exposure to mosquitoes.

In some cases, the mosquitoes caught in the traps are tested for the presence of specific pathogens, such as the Zika virus. The species of mosquito is also reported from these tests to help inform preventive efforts. The National Environment Agency combines the data it gets from clinics and mosquito traps with a variety of other relevant data—population demographics, temperature, humidity, vegetation index, the age of buildings, and the number of units in buildings—and puts them into a temporal model that predicts the likelihood of outbreaks (Shi et al., 2016). The model did a good job of predicting a dengue outbreak in 2013, Ng said, but it predicted an outbreak in 2016 that did not materialize. In retrospection, this miss was likely due to the unusually high heat from El Niño that year. A prediction of an outbreak in 2022 was borne out, although it arrived several weeks earlier than predicted. On a more granular scale, the data are put into a random forest algorithm to predict which areas in Singapore are at the highest risk (Ong et al., 2018). Those predictions have proven to be quite accurate as well, Ng said; for instance, nearly 90 percent of large clusters (10 cases or more) occurred in areas that had been identified as high risk in the model.

In addition to predicting outbreaks and knowing where to allocate resources, Ng described how the surveillance tools developed by the National Environment Agency help in evaluating the effectiveness of their control measures and in estimating the economic impact of those measures. The control measures can calculate how much money is saved in health care costs and to what extent human productivity and efforts are conserved, which provides an economic justification of the funds spent on surveillance and prevention.

DIAGNOSTICS FOR ARBOVIRUS MITIGATION

Boeras spoke about how diagnostics can be used for arbovirus mitigation, what effective diagnostic tools are available, and how widely they can be deployed. She began by discussing what has been achieved and what still needs more attention in the three different ways that diagnostics are used: to prepare for an epidemic, to prevent an epidemic, and to respond to an epidemic.

In the case of preparing for an epidemic, she said, what has already been done includes carrying out landscape reviews of what is available and what is in the pipeline, determining target product profiles, and evaluating diagnostic tests through networks of expert laboratories. What is still lacking, she said, is the creation of a framework for specimen and data sharing, the promotion of local manufacturing to improve access to tests, and the education of care providers and communities to raise awareness of these various issues. With regard to the prevention, there has been significant accomplishments in the development of diagnostics for early and rapid case detections and also diagnostics to support deployment of transmission prevention measures. On the other hand, Boeras said, there is still insufficient investment in real-time surveillance, particularly for diagnostics with connectivity functions that could allow for better, real-time use of surveillance data. Finally, in terms of diagnostics for response, Boeras pointed out that current tools can already be used to carry out rapid assessments of the extent of outbreaks and genomic sequencing when diagnostic testing is available. Areas where more work is needed include the stockpiling of diagnostics equipment and material, engaging with the community and raising awareness, and aligning use of diagnostics with vaccine research and development, she said.

Boeras offered some background details on how the diagnosis of a viral disease such as dengue is carried out. With primary infection, the virus enters the bloodstream (viraemia), triggering the production of the antibodies immunoglobulin M (IgM) and immunoglobulin G (IgG). If this is a secondary infection, the level of IgG will increase sharply from an already elevated level, while IgM will only have a small increase from the near-baseline level after the end of the primary infection. In 2010, Boeras said, Peeling and colleagues examined this pattern to understand how it translates into diagnostics, particularly for patient management and disease surveillance. A variety of diagnostic tools are available for clinicians to confirm infection during the acute phase: virus isolation, nucleic acid detection, antigen detection, and, in some cases, it is possible to look for IgM seroconversion and an approximately fourfold rise in IgG titers (i.e., the IgG concentration). Boeras noted the benefit of serology testing in public health surveillance, where a population baseline of IgM can be established so that an increased number of IgM-positive individuals or higher IgM titers could indicate a potential outbreak. Confirmation of the outbreak could be done by using reverse transcription polymerase chain reaction (RT-PCR) to look for viral messenger RNA (mRNA).

However, there remain challenges in carrying out serological diagnostics of emerging arboviruses, Boeras remarked. A 2021 review examined the performance of readily available, commonly used commercial antibody and antigen tests and identified five categories of challenges (Fischer et al., 2021). The first is the inherent limitation(s) from how the intrinsic properties of different test formats limit their performance, such as the differences in sensitivity or specificity between an enzyme-linked immunosorbent assay (ELISA) and a rapid diagnostic test. A second challenge is that the timing of a serological test is crucial—exactly when a patient presents symptoms can significantly affect test results. Third, individual infection histories can also affect diagnostic test performance, and a major issue is referred to as "original antigenic sin"; this is when the patient may react to a new infection when they were previously exposed to a closely related antigen by mounting a response to the first antigen rather than the new antigen (Vatti et al., 2017). "So for example," Boeras explained, "if your first infection with a flavivirus is dengue, and then you got infected with Zika, your antibody response would still be higher for dengue than for Zika." In that case, the only way to correctly diagnose the Zika infection would be with RT-PCR. One problem, she continued, is that most pregnant women in resource-limited settings tend to delay seeking medical care and the window for PCR positivity may pass before they visit a clinic, thus making it very difficult to diagnose a Zika infection. This is a major problem because of the effects that Zika can have on a fetus. A fourth challenge is the global mixing of antigenically related viruses. Since dengue, Zika, and chikungunya may all be circulating in a population at the same time, it can be difficult to know what virus or viruses a person who tests positive was exposed to. The final challenges are polyclonal B cell activation and environmental factors.

Returning to the challenge posed by the different performances of different tests, Boeras highlighted that these serological tests show a broad range of sensitivities and specificities. For example, the IgM ELISA test for chikungunya has reasonable sensitivity and high specificity, but the IgM rapid diagnostic test (RDT) for chikungunya has extremely low sensitivity. The IgM RDT for dengue and the IgM ELISA test for Zika both have a high median specificity, but the range of specificity values from different studies is very large, indicating that cross reactivity between the two viruses may be a problem. This situation is complicated by the fact that the sensitivities of the different tests vary over time, and they do not always vary in the same way, Boeras said.

Using different tests together in reaching a diagnosis may be one way to address these challenges, Boeras suggested. A 2016 study by Hunsperger and colleagues used paired serum samples from 1,234 laboratory-confirmed dengue patients to show that over 90 percent of the primary and secondary dengue cases were accurately identified by using either IgM ELISA with RT-PCR or IgM ELISA with the NS1 antigen ELISA. Boeras also described recent work to develop effective diagnostic tests for Zika. As part of this effort, and in response to the Zika outbreak, UNICEF and the U.S. Agency for International Development established an advanced purchase commitment mechanism aimed at incentivizing companies to develop assays that were more accurate and accessible, with a specific focus on serological rapid diagnostic tests. Once a test was validated, UNICEF was committed to procuring millions of them for countries to use as part of arbovirus surveillance programs.

Boeras's group was involved in evaluating the tests submitted to this program, and she described the multisite approach they used. They conducted quick pass or fail assessments on three RDTs, two of which had satisfactory performance to progress to full lab-based evaluations (Boeras et al., 2022). Then in conjunction with partners, such as the Institute Pasteur Dakar in Senegal, these assays were evaluated for feasibility in the field. There were nine testing facilities in two regions, one with the highest known Zika transmission rates in Senegal and another with one of the lowest. A key feature to the program, Boeras said, was that the researchers engaged the community, including leaders and health authorities. Health care workers who participated in this evaluation program received trainings over 2–3 days and reported back on their user experience, revealing insights such as that RDTs were especially useful for screening of pregnant women because they can be used at remote sites, Boeras said. Most of the health care workers agreed to integrate the RDTs into routine services for pregnant women. For surveillance, the workers preferred to use multiplex panels that would test for Zika as well as for chikungunya, dengue, and yellow fever, but they concluded that the single test was better suited for the point-of-care diagnosis at district-level health centers where pregnant women were presenting.

In summary, Boeras shared that dengue diagnostics are now on the WHO list of essential diagnostics but there are opportunities for continued improvement. While RDTs exist for point-of-care diagnosis, "we are still looking at external quality assurance programs for these," she said. There is ongoing work to develop multiplex tests for patient management and surveillance, and to ensure existing multiplex tests are broadly affordable and accessible. More specific antigen or molecular detection tests are also needed to confirm Zika infection for use in patient management at the point of care. Ongoing research and development can be directed toward creating more rapid but less expensive multiplex molecular tests that can distinguish among febrile illnesses caused by the dengue, chikungunya, and Zika viruses, Boeras said. There is also a need for more specific and high-throughput antibody detection tests that can be used on a population basis for surveillance of arbovirus infection and for epidemiological studies. Finally, connectivity capabilities that can link data between diagnostic laboratories and point-of-care test devices could provide early warnings for infectious disease outbreaks as well as timely information for disease control and prevention programs, which in turn would increase the efficiency of health care systems and improve patient outcomes.

DISCUSSION

Speaking to Ng, Scott asked about key considerations for other regions that may want to set up a dengue control program similar to the one in Singapore. "Environment management is one of the most important things when it comes to vector control programs," she answered. Singapore's program not only focused on dengue control, but also included efforts to keep the city clean and to relocate residents from slum housing to high-rise apartments. These efforts worked together synergistically to first eliminate malaria (Singapore was declared malaria-free by WHO in 1989) and then to address *Aedes aegypti* and dengue. A second important factor, she added, is social mobilization. The Singapore government worked to get the community involved so that removing water containers become as much a part of life as brushing teeth. Cultivating such habits was crucial, Ng stressed.

Harris asked Ng about how residents are encouraged to pay attention to health alerts in Singapore. Public education will reach maybe 90 percent of the population, Ng replied, but there will still be 5 to 10 percent who are not as vigilant, and, unfortunately, the vector control of dengue is only as strong as the weakest link. "If you have a block of flats and you have one person breeding mosquitoes, the whole block is at risk." Singapore has a system of civil penalties to address this gap in societal vigilance. Health officers will conduct home visits to check for potential mosquito breeding sites, and a person who is found with active mosquito breeding in their home will be fined.

One attendee asked Rojas about the dashboard she had described in her talk. Noting that the quality of the dashboard will depend on the quality of the data provided at the local level, where it has always been a struggle to get high-quality data, she asked what role WHO or other large multinational organizations play in the development of easy-to-use tools that could be used on the ground. WHO has been working with its regional offices to figure out which tools are needed by different countries and to determine the best ways to report the data and the analyses, Rojas said. "We're a little bit behind with some of the regions, such as the African region, because right now they are starting to see arboviruses as a threat," she said. Malaria was the biggest arboviral threat in the African region, but efforts to tackle this have paid off and malaria cases have been declining, while non-malaria arboviral disease cases are going up. "And now, with the capacities that were built for COVID, they are realizing that they have more arbovirus transmission than what they thought they had. So, with them we are now going to create a parallel surveillance system." WHO will try to include arboviruses in the DHIS2, a tool for reporting malaria and other diseases, which has been used in Africa as well as in the western Pacific and the Caribbean. Rojas concluded, "we've been working with the regions at trying to address, at the local level where the data is generated, which is the best tool to gather the data on arboviruses." The goal is to build a surveillance system that can provide data not just on malaria or HIV but also on all infectious diseases, including arboviral diseases. In addition, Rojas agreed with another attendee's comment that malaria or arboviral disease funding should not be framed as opposing each other another. "What we need to do is to put arboviral diseases into the top level of discussion, as PAHO has done it with all the resolutions throughout the years," she said, "and do a similar exercise with the other countries, even bringing it to the World Health Assembly to have the political commitment to have continuous funding."

Asked about communicating genomic surveillance, Faria mentioned the numerous training workshops he hosted that were attended by PAHO and Brazilian Ministry of Health colleagues. Faria said that he tried to always bring stakeholders to the workshops, so that the students he mentored could see what was expected from the genomic data from the stakeholders' perspective. "I think that involvement with the stakeholders is really important because it also allows us to target a little bit more the questions that we need to address."

REFERENCES

Aik, J., Z. W. Neo, J. Rajarethinam, K. Chio, W. M. Lam, and L.-C. Ng. 2019. The effectiveness of inspections on reported mosquito larval habitats in households: A case–control study. *PLOS Neglected Tropical Diseases* 13(6):e0007492.

Boeras, D., C. T. Diagne, J. L. Pelegrino, M. Grandadam, V. Duong, P. Dussart, P. Brey, D. Ruiz, M. Adati, A. Wilder-Smith, A. K. Falconar, C. M. Romero, M. Guzman, N. Hasanin, A. Sall, and R. W. Peeling. 2022. Evaluation of Zika rapid tests as aids for clinical diagnosis and epidemic preparedness. *eClinicalMedicine* 49:101478.

Faria, N. R., J. Quick, I.M. Claro, J. Thézé, J. G. de Jesus, M. Giovanetti, M. U. G. Kraemer, S. C. Hill, A. Black, A. C. da Costa, L. C. Franco, S. P. Silva, C.-H. Wu, J. Raghwani, S. Cauchemez, L. du Plessis, M. P. Verotti, W. K. de Oliveira, E. H. Carmo, G. E. Coelho, A. C. F. S. Santelli, L. C. Vinhal, C. M. Henriques, J. T. Simpson, M. Loose, K. G. Andersen, N. D. Grubaugh, S. Somasekar, C. Y. Chiu, J. E. Muñoz-Medina, C. R. Gonzalez-Bonilla, C. F. Arias, L. L. Lewis-Ximenez, S. A. Baylis, A. O. Chieppe, S. F. Aguiar, C. A. Fernandes, P. S. Lemos, B. L. S. Nascimento, H. A. O. Monteiro, I. C. Siqueira, M. G. de Queiroz, T. R. de Souza, J. F. Bezerra, M. R. Lemos, G. F. Pereira, D. Loudal, L. C. Moura, R. Dhalia, R. F. França, T. Magalhães, E. T. Marques Jr, T. Jaenisch, G. L. Wallau, M. C. de Lima, V. Nascimento, E. M. de Cerqueira, M. M. de Lima, D. L. Mascarenhas, J. P. Moura Neto, A. S. Levin, T. R. Tozetto-Mendoza, S. N. Fonseca, M. C. Mendes-Correa, F. P. Milagres, A. Segurado, E. C. Holmes, A. Rambaut, T. Bedford, M. R. T. Nunes, E. C. Sabino, L. C. J. Alcantara, N. J. Loman, and O. G. Pybus. 2017. Establishment and cryptic transmission of Zika virus in Brazil and the Americas. *Nature* 546:406–410.

Faria, N. R., M. U. G. Kraemer, S. C. Hill, J. Goes de Jesus, R. S. Aguiar, F. C. M. Iani, J. Xavier, J. Quick, L. du Plessis, S. Dellicour, J. Thézé, R. D. O. Carvalho, G. Baele, C.-H. Wu, P. P. Silveira, M. B. Arruda, M. A. Pereira, G. C. Pereira, J. Lourenço, U. Obolski, L. Abade, T. I. Vasylyeva, M. Giovanetti, D. Yi, D. J. Weiss, G. R. W. Wint, F. M. Shearer, S. Funk, B. Nikolay, V. Fonseca, T.E.R. Adelino, M. A. A. Oliveira, M. V. F. Silva, L. Sacchetto, P. O. Figueiredo, I. M. Rezende, E.M. Mello, R.F.C. Said, D.A. Santos, M. L. Ferraz, M. G. Brito, L. F. Santana, M. T. Menezes, R. M. Brindeiro, A. Tanuri, F.C.P. dos Santos, M. S. Cunha, J. S. Nogueira, I. M. Rocco, A. C. da Costa, C. S. V. Komninakis, V. Azevedo, A. O. Chieppe, E. S. M. Araujo, M. C. L. Mendonça, C. C. dos Santos, C. D. dos Santos, A. M. Mares-Guia, R. M. R. Nogueira, P. C. Sequeira, R. G. Abreu, M. H. O. Garcia, A. L. Abreu, O. Okumoto, E. G. Kroon, C. F. C. de Albuquerque, K. Lewandowski, S. T. Pullan, M. Carroll, T. de Oliveira, E. C. Sabino, R. P. Souza, M. A. Suchard, P. Lemey, G. S. Trindade, B. P. Drumond, A. M. B. Filippis, N. J. Loman, S. Cauchemez, L. C. J. Alcantara, and O. G. Pybus. 2018. Genomic and epidemiological monitoring of yellow fever virus transmission potential. *Science* 361(6405):894–899. https://doi.org/10.1126/science.aat7115

Fischer, C., W. K. Jo, V. Haage, A. Moreira-Soto, E. F. de Oliveira Filho, and J. F. Drexler. 2021. Challenges towards serologic diagnostics of emerging arboviruses. *Clinical Microbiology and Infection* 27(9):1221–1229.

Grubaugh, N. D. J. T. Ladner, M. U. G. Kraemer, G. Dudas, A. L. Tan, K. Gangavarapu, M. R. Wiley, S. White, J. Thézé, D. M. Magnani, K. Prieto, D. Reyes, A. M. Bingham, L. M. Paul, R. Robles-Sikisaka, G. Oliveira, D. Pronty, C. M. Barcellona, H. C. Metsky, M. L. Baniecki, K. G. Barnes, B. Chak, C. A. Freije, A. Gladden-Young, A. Gnirke, C. Luo, B. MacInnis, C. B. Matranga, D. J. Park, J. Qu, S. F. Schaffner, C. Tomkins-Tinch, K. L. West, S. M. Winnicki, S. Wohl, N. L. Yozwiak, J. Quick, J. R. Fauver, K. Khan, S. E. Brent, R. C. Reiner Jr., P. N. Lichtenberger, M. J. Ricciardi, V. K. Bailey, D. I. Watkins, M. R. Cone, E. W. Kopp IV, K. N. Hogan, A. C. Cannons, R. Jean, A. J. Monaghan, R. F. Garry, N. J. Loman, N. R. Faria, M. C. Porcelli, C. Vasquez, E. R. Nagle, D. A. T. Cummings, D. Stanek, A. Rambaut, M. Sanchez-Lockhart, P. C. Sabeti, L. D. Gillis, S. F. Michael, T. Bedford, O. G. Pybus, S. Isern, G. Palacios, and K. G. Andersen. 2017. Genomic epidemiology reveals multiple introductions of Zika virus into the United States. *Nature* 546:401–405.

Hill, S. C., J. Vasconcelos, Z. Neto, D. Jandondo, L. Zé-Zé, R. S. Aguiar, J. Xavier, J. Thézé, M. Mirandela, A. L. Micolo Cândido, F. Vaz, C. d. S. Sebastião, C.-H. Wu, M. U. G. Kraemer, A. Melo, B. L. F. Schamber-Reis, G. S. de Azevedo, A. Tanuri, L. M. Higa, C. Clemente, S. P. da Silva, D. da Silva Candido, I. M. Claro, D. Quibuco, C. Domingos, B. Pocongo, A. G. Watts, K. Khan, L. C. J. Alcantara, E. C. Sabino, E. Lackritz, O. G. Pybus, M.-J. Alves, J. Afonso, and N. R. Faria. 2019. Emergence of the Asian lineage of Zika virus in Angola: an outbreak investigation. *The Lancet Infectious Diseases* 19(10): 1138–1147. https://doi.org/10.1016/S1473-3099(19)30293-2

Ho, S. H., J. T. Lim, J. Ong, H. C. Hapuarachchi, S. Sim, and L.-C. Ng. 2023. Singapore's 5 decades of dengue prevention and control—Implications for global dengue control. *PLOS Neglected Tropical Diseases* 17(6):e001140.

Hunsperger, E. A., J. Muñoz-Jordán, M. Beltran, C. Colón, J. Carrión, J. Vazquez, L. N. Acosta, J. F. Medina-Izquierdo, K. Horiuchi, B. J. Biggerstaff, and H. S. Margolis. 2016. Performance of dengue diagnostic tests in a single-specimen diagnostic algorithm. *Journal of Infectious Diseases* 214(6):836–844.

Ng, L.-C., L. K. Tan, C. H. Tan, S. S. Tan, H. C. Hapuarachchi, K. Y. Pok, Y. L. Lai, S. G. Lam-Phua, G. Bucht, R. T. Lin, Y. S. Leo, B. H. Tan, H. K. Han, P. L. Ooi, L. James, and S. P. Khoo. 2009. Entomologic and virologic investigation of chikungunya, Singapore. *Emerging Infectious Diseases* 15(8):1243–1249.

Ong, J., X. Liu, J. Rajarethinam, S. Y. Kok, S. Liang, C. S. Tang, A. R. Cook, L.-C. Ng, and G. Yap. 2018. Mapping dengue risk in Singapore using random forest. *PLOS Neglected Tropical Diseases* 12(6):e0006587.

Ong, J., J. Aik, and L.-C. Ng. 2021. Short report: Adult *Aedes* abundance and risk of dengue transmission. *PLOS Neglected Tropical Diseases* 15(6):e0009475.

Peeling, R. W., H. Artsob, J. L. Pelegrino, P. Buchy, M. J. Cardosa, S. Devi, D. A. Enria, J. Farrar, D. F. Gubler, M. G. Guzman, S. B. Halstead, E. Hunsperger, S. Kliks, H. S. Margolis, C. M. Nathanson, V. C. Nguyen, N. Rizzo, S. Vázquez, and S. Yoksan. 2010. Evaluation of diagnostic tests: Dengue. *Nature Reviews Microbiology* 8(12 Suppl):S30–S38.

Rajarethinam, J., L. W. Ang, J. Ong, J. Ycasas, H. C. Hapuarachchi, G. Yap, C. S. Chong, Y. L. Lai, J. Cutter, D. Ho, V. Lee, and L.-C. Ng. 2018. Dengue in Singapore from 2004 to 2016: Cyclical epidemic patterns dominated by serotypes 1 and 2. *American Journal of Tropical Medicine and Hygiene* 99(1):204–210.

Sayers, E. W., M. Cavanaugh, K. Clark, K. D. Pruitt, S. T. Sherry, L. Yankie, and I. Karsch-Mizrachi. 2023. GenBank 2023 update. *Nucleic Acids Research* 51(D1):D141–D144. https://doi.org/10.1093/nar/gkac1012.

Shi, Y., X. Liu, S. Y. Kok, J. Rajarethinam, S. Liang, G. Yap, C. S. Chong, K. S. Lee, S. S. Tan, C. K. Chin, A. Lo, W. Kong, L.-C. Ng, and A. R. Cook. 2016. Three-month teal-time dengue forecast models: An early warning system for outbreak alerts and policy decision support in Singapore. *Environmental Health Perspectives* 124(9):1369–1375.

Sim, S., L.-C. Ng., S. W. Lindsay, and A. L. Wilson. 2020. A greener vision for vector control: The example of the Singapore dengue control programme. *PLOS Neglected Tropical Diseases* 14(8):e0008428.

Vatti, A., D. M. Monsalve, Y. Pacheco, C. Chang, J. M. Anaya, and M. E. Gershwin. 2017. Original antigenic sin: A comprehensive review. *Journal of Autoimunolgy* 83:12–21.

4

Response to Arboviral Threats

Highlights

- An ideal vaccine for arboviruses would be a single-dose vaccine that provides long-lasting protection, has a high safety profile, and is produced with cutting-edge technology that avoids the challenges of scaling up with traditional manufacturing. (Paz-Bailey)
- Alternative licensing pathways are needed for some vaccines. (Paz-Bailey)
- Vaccine hesitancy can be very damaging to the implementation of vaccine programs. (Paz-Bailey)
- History has shown that vector control works, but until recently there has been relatively little evidence demonstrating which types of vector control are most effective for preventing infection and/or disease in which situations. More research on the public health value of vector control is needed. (Scott)
- Several innovative vector-control techniques have been developed in recent years; these should continue to be tested and, where warranted, put to work. (Scott)
- The best approach to controlling arbovirus infections will likely involve a combination of individual methods. This could include combinations of different vector-control strategies or combining vector control with a vaccine. (Scott)

continued

- The Pan American Health Organization (PAHO) has established a collaborative surveillance program in which countries provide data that PAHO aggregates, analyzes, and makes available back to the countries to assist in their arbovirus prevention and control efforts. (dos Santos)
- Models can be used for various purposes, including improving scientific understanding of arbovirus outbreaks, estimating various epidemiological parameters that cannot be measured directly, predicting the consequences of various intervention choices, and forecasting the timing and behavior of outbreaks. (Brady)
- It is important for modelers not only to work on improving their models but also to collaborate with health officials and others so that those models can be put to effective use. (Brady)

NOTE: These points were made by the individual workshop speakers/participants identified above. They are not intended to reflect a consensus among workshop participants.

The workshop's third session, moderated by Ann M. Powers, associate director for science at the Centers for Disease Control and Prevention, was devoted to the various ways that researchers, public health officials, and others have responded to arbovirus threats. The types of responses in the session included disease and vector surveillance, vector control, vaccines, and modeling. Gabriela Paz-Bailey, chief of the Dengue Branch, Division of Vector-Borne Diseases at the Centers for Disease Control and Prevention, gave an overview of current arbovirus vaccines. Thomas W. Scott, a distinguished professor of mosquito-transmitted disease ecology and epidemiology at the University of California, Davis, spoke about types of vector control. Thais dos Santos, regional advisor for surveillance and control of arboviral diseases at the Pan American Health Organization (PAHO), discussed arboviral diseases surveillance and integrated surveillance in the Americas. And Oliver Brady, an associate professor at the London School of Hygiene and Tropical Medicine, described the various ways that models can be used in arbovirus surveillance and control. A question-and-answer session followed the four presentations.

ARBOVIRUS VACCINES

Paz-Bailey began by providing brief overviews of the vaccines that have been developed for chikungunya, Japanese encephalitis, Zika, West Nile virus, yellow fever, and dengue with a focus on the specific challenges encountered in each of the vaccines' development. Then she offered a list of lessons that could be gleaned from the experiences with these vaccines, focusing on the idea that these lessons could help the public health sector be better prepared to deal with the next arbovirus pandemic.

Chikungunya

VLA1553, the first-ever chikungunya vaccine to be licensed, is a single-dose vaccine manufactured by the company Valneva. It was licensed by the U.S. Food and Drug Administration under accelerated approval for adults aged 18 years and older; that approval is based on the persistence of neutralizing antibodies at up to 6 months after administration of the vaccine. Recent 2-year follow-up data show that 97 percent of those vaccinated maintained antibody titers, Paz-Bailey said. The vaccine is under review by the European Medicines Agency, while the World Health Organization (WHO) is at the initial stages of considering recommendations for global use. Importantly, she added, the Coalition for Epidemic Preparedness Innovations has provided funding for VLA1553 and other chikungunya vaccines to ensure that low- and middle-income countries have access to the vaccines.

Other chikungunya vaccines are in phase 3 trials, Paz-Bailey said, either completing the trials or in the middle of them. The first is a single-dose, virus-like vaccine manufactured by Bavarian Nordic, and the second is BBV87, manufactured in collaboration by International Vaccine Institute in South Korea and Bharat Biotech in India. It is an inactivated whole-virus vaccine, administered with a two-dose primary series.

The chikungunya vaccines face various challenges. The phase 3 trials provide data on immunogenicity and safety but not on efficacy, Paz-Bailey said. Since there is no way to predict where the outbreaks will occur, antibody titers are used as a correlate of protection; however, this endpoint has not been validated against efficacy data. Long-term protection for the vaccines is also still unknown, which hinders the accelerated approval process that requires data from post-licensure studies. Finally, the ideal implementation strategy remains unknown. Given that the outbreaks can be very localized and completed within a couple of months, it is challenging to respond quickly enough to make a major difference.

Japanese Encephalitis

Next Paz-Bailey spoke about vaccines for Japanese encephalitis, which generally affects humans in rural areas who live and work close to pigs. Vaccines for the disease have been available for decades, with most endemic countries now having vaccination programs. Gavi, the Vaccine Alliance, has expanded the use of WHO-prequalified vaccines for Japanese encephalitis.

SA 14-14-2 is a live attenuated vaccine developed in China that is available at low cost to low- and middle-income countries. Many manufacturers have developed inactivated Vero cell culture–based production and live attenuated vaccines, which are easier to manufacture. Ixiaro is the only Japanese encephalitis vaccine licensed and available in the United States (Vannice et al., 2021). The challenges facing the Japanese encephalitis vaccine are representative of those facing other arbovirus vaccines, Paz-Bailey said. They include predicting outbreaks, when transmission will occur, and producing enough vaccines to meet the global supply needs.

Zika

Many Zika vaccine candidates are in clinical trials, including a purified inactivated vaccine that has shown to be immunogenic after two doses, a live attenuated virus, and a chimeric measles vaccine that expresses some proteins of Zika. A DNA vaccine for Zika is currently in phase 2B trials in several sites in the United States and Latin America. Among the challenges facing Zika vaccines, congenital Zika syndrome may develop from infection at any point during pregnancy, which means that a Zika vaccine must provide protection against infection, Paz-Bailey said. Many other challenges exist: Cases have declined, so it is impossible to carry out phase 3 trials to assess efficacy, and there is no validated immune correlate of protection. Furthermore, the small number of participants in the phase 2 trials is not enough to allow the detection of infrequent but severe outcomes, such as Guillain-Barré syndrome. Ethical issues arise in conducting efficacy trials in pregnant women. Paz-Bailey shared that there are concerns about the interaction between the Zika virus and dengue with the possibility that vaccinating seronegative individuals who have not been exposed to dengue could increase their chances of contracting severe disease if they are later exposed to dengue. Also, the efficacy of the Zika vaccine may depend on an individual's dengue exposure or serostatus. Finally, Paz-Bailey said, alternative licensing pathways are needed that could consider efficacy from human challenge models and extrapolate protection from animal models to humans.

West Nile Virus

Concerning the West Nile virus, Paz-Bailey said that several veterinary vaccines have been licensed for horses, but no human vaccine has been authorized. Several vaccine candidates have been evaluated in human trials, but none have progressed beyond phase 1 or phase 2. All these trials found minimal adverse events, and most found favorable immunogenicity. Concerning the challenges facing West Nile vaccines, the sporadic and unpredictable nature of the virus makes it hard to plan efficacy trials. Severe disease is more common in those older than 50 years of age and with comorbidities, and there are concerns about vaccines causing adverse events for those in this group. Also, there is no consensus on what the trial endpoints should be, whether preventing neuroinvasive disease, preventing all diseases, or preventing infection. The endpoint chosen will affect the feasibility of conducting phase 3 trials. West Nile virus vaccination programs are expensive, and their cost-effectiveness is not clear. Finally, as with Zika vaccines, Paz-Bailey said, alternative licensing pathways are needed for West Nile virus vaccines that would consider approval based on immune protection in animal models and immunological markers.

Yellow Fever

Turning to yellow fever vaccines, Paz-Bailey said that a live attenuated yellow fever vaccine, 17D, has been applied safely and effectively for more than 80 years. One dose of the vaccine can generate long-lasting antibodies, and WHO no longer recommends a booster dose after 10 years. There have been no formal efficacy studies to determine how well the vaccine protects against specific adverse health outcomes, she said, but its effectiveness has been demonstrated through its use in practice in endemic areas and in laboratory workers. Fractional doses have been shown to be safe and effective, with one-fifth of a dose resulting in comparable protection for 10 years, so fractional doses have been used as a temporary solution for vaccine shortages. Several vaccine candidates for yellow fever are under development, with three of them now in clinical trials, but these vaccines would require multiple doses to achieve the same level of protective, long-lasting immunity that the current vaccine achieves (Montalvo Zurbia-Flores et al., 2022).

Speaking of the vaccine's challenges, Paz-Bailey said that although adverse events are rare, there is a higher risk of occurrence in persons 60 years of age and older. The vaccine is contraindicated for pregnant and lactating women, infants under 6 months, persons older than 60 years, and those with severe immunodeficiency or hypersensitivity to eggs. Vaccine manufacturing is difficult to scale up because the vaccine is produced using traditional chicken-embryo methods, and even with six manufacturers globally, shortages of the vaccine still occur.

Dengue

For dengue, the Dengvaxia vaccine produced by Sanofi is a tetravalent, live attenuated vaccine. The vaccine requires three doses administered 6 months apart, so people need a full year before they are fully vaccinated. One problem with the vaccine is that it increases the risk of hospitalizations among children who have not been exposed to dengue virus before, i.e., those who are seronegative. Thus, it is recommended to be used only among seropositive individuals. A laboratory test to assess the dengue serostatus must be done before administering the vaccine, which makes it very challenging to implement.[1] A second vaccine, QDENGA, produced by Takeda is a tetravalent live attenuated vaccine. It is administered in two doses given 3 months apart, and its efficacy is 61 percent against disease and 84 percent against hospitalization. In those who are seropositive, it protects against all four serotypes, while in seronegative individuals it protects against dengue-1 and dengue-2 but not against dengue-3, and there is insufficient data for dengue-4. WHO recommends that it be given to children 6–16 years in high-transmission areas, irrespective of their serostatus. A third vaccine, TV003 from Merck and the Butantan Institute, is live attenuated and requires one dose. Phase 3 trial results in Brazil found that after 2 years of follow-up, the efficacy against symptomatic disease was 89 percent for seropositive and 73 percent for seronegative.

A major challenge for dengue vaccines, Paz-Bailey said, is that they need to be four vaccines in one since they must provide protection against all four of the serotypes to avoid antibody-dependent enhancement. There is also no clear correlate of protection, and a longer period of observation following vaccination is necessary to make sure there is no increased risk of severe disease and hospitalization.

Lessons

In closing, Paz-Bailey offered several lessons. An ideal vaccine for arboviruses would be a single-dose vaccine that provides long-lasting protection, has a high safety profile, and is produced with cutting-edge technology to avoid the challenges of scaling up with traditional manufacturing. Vaccine development acceleration technologies are available, but funding has been a major obstacle for the progress of novel vaccines. It will be important to bring together public health institutions, governments, pharmaceutical companies, and nongovernmental organizations to establish priorities and settle on a united purpose, "as we are hoping we can achieve during this meeting," Paz-Bailey added. Vaccine hesitancy can be very challenging to the implementation of vaccine programs, and it is something that should be addressed, noted Paz-Bailey. Finally, alternative licensing pathways could be prioritized for some vaccines.

---

[1] Production of the Dengvaxia vaccine has been discontinued by the manufacturer, and available doses will expire in August 2026. See https://www.cdc.gov/dengue/vaccine/index.html (accessed June 14, 2024).

VECTOR CONTROL

When vector control is done properly, it prevents disease, Scott said at the beginning of his remarks. This has been shown many times over, as with yellow-fever prevention efforts during the construction of the Panama Canal and in the hemisphere-wide campaign to eradicate *Aedes aegypti* from the Americas. More recently, programs in the 1970s and 1980s in Singapore and in the 1980s and 1990s in Cuba used adult and larval control to reduce dengue.

Despite these successes, vector control has not always been effective. Several years ago, experts realized that the evidence base for vector control tools that have been used for decades is too often not strong. Rather than including epidemiological outcomes demonstrating the impact on human disease or infection, most trials in the past were limited to entomological outcomes. A 2015 paper by Anne Wilson et al. addressed the design of phase 3 clinical trials for the assessment of vector control and concluded that the public health information such trials produced could enhance innovation for vector-borne disease control. After that, the Vector Control Advisory Group at WHO developed a detailed document explaining how to carry out a vector-control phase 3 trial (WHO, 2017). Many of the tools that have been used for the last 50 years have not been evaluated, Scott noted. However, Scott noted that many new tools are being evaluated in well-designed phase 3 trials, which proves helpful in developing public health policy.

Scott described the current interventions used for vector control and the innovative methods now being developed. The current interventions can be grouped into two categories: interventions that target immature mosquitoes and those that target adult mosquitoes. Getting rid of immature mosquitoes involves a combination of source reduction: getting rid of the sites where mosquito larvae develop and treatment of the sites to kill the larva or prevent them from maturing into adults. These site treatments can be carried out with insect growth regulators, chemical insecticides, biological treatments, or predation. Interventions for adult mosquitoes include space-spraying from trucks and aircraft, personal protection with topical repellants, and indoor residual spraying. These interventions can be either reactive or proactive. Reactive interventions are generally carried out in response to an increase in cases and use insecticides aimed at adult mosquitoes to quickly lower the number of adult mosquitoes in an area. Proactive interventions are intended to block outbreaks before they begin and generally combine methods aimed at controlling both adult and immature mosquitoes. The proactive approaches, Scott said, deserve greater emphasis and are the direction that the field needs to go.

Scott divided innovations in arbovirus vector control into two groups: innovations that are in development and innovations that are in or have completed phase 3 trials. The in-development techniques include larval control with fungi and autodissemination; population suppression with such methods as *Wolbachia*, sterile insects, toxic sugar baits, and the release of insects with a dominant lethal gene; population modification with homing endonuclease genes; CRISPR-Cas9 gene-driven systems to create virus-resistant mosquito strains; and population reduction with sterile females or reduced female survival. Techniques that have gone through phase 3 trials include a population modification approach by the World Mosquito Program, which involves introducing *Wolbachia* bacteria into a mosquito population. Wolbachia infection in mosquitoes confers resistance to infection and, therefore, reduces virus transmission and human disease. A phase 3 trial of the technique in Indonesia led to an almost 80 percent reduction in virologically confirmed dengue, "which is really a remarkable outcome," Scott said. The program is now carrying out a second trial in Brazil.

A trial in Peru tested spatial repellants, which are chemicals released into the air that interfere with mosquitoes biting humans. The results were promising, according to Scott, with a 34 percent reduction in Zika and dengue infections in humans. A second trial of the repellant began in late 2023 in Sri Lanka. Recently, Scott added, S. C. Johnson, the manufacturer of the product, has come out with a new product called Guardian, which the company claims will be effective for 1 year. This would be a major improvement, Scott explained, as the product used in the Peru trials had to be reapplied every 2 weeks, while the one in the Sri Lanka trials must be swapped out once a month. Another effective current innovation, Scott said, is targeted indoor residual spraying. An initial trial in Australia, where the targeted indoor residual spraying was combined with contact tracing, reduced dengue infection by 90 percent. Results from a trial now going on in Mexico should be available within the next year.

Looking to the future, Scott identified Africa as one area of growing concern for arbovirus infections. In the next 50 to 70 years, there will be a huge increase in the construction of urban environments around the world, and much of that will take place in Africa. "There's an opportunity there for *Aedes* mosquitoes to get into those environments and create a public health disaster," he said. According to a recent WHO assessment, many African countries have limited programs dedicated to *Aedes* vector surveillance, a lack of surveillance for insecticide resistance in *Aedes* mosquitoes, and no regular training session for specialists in vector control and surveillance of *Aedes* vectors. Much of the entomological expertise in Africa today is related to malaria and not so much with *Aedes*, Scott said, and this could be a growing problem in the future. He pointed to multiple resources that could help address this issue in Africa, such as the Global Arbovirus Initiative and *Global Vector Control Response 2017–2030*. There is also the West African *Aedes* Surveillance Network, which was formed in 2017

(Dadzie et al., 2022). A related publication by Roiz et al. (2018), offers a systematic, step-by-step process for the comprehensive control of *Aedes*-borne infections.

Speaking briefly about tick-borne disease, Scott pointed to three publications that discussed the best ways to protect people from tick-borne diseases (Eisen, 2020; Keesing et al., 2022; Stafford, 2004). These publications indicate that like mosquito control, many methods of tick control have not been evaluated for their public health value. However, there is growing interest in assessing the effectiveness of techniques to better inform the public health policies that are being developed.

In closing, Scott offered his thoughts on what people in the field should focus on most going forward. First, he said, it will be important to figure out which of the long-standing methods are effective in preventing human infection and disease and which should not be recommended any more. Noting the difficulty of getting funding for clinical trials of such accepted methods, he suggested finding alternative ways to test their effectiveness. Second, the innovation in vector control needs to continue. Creators of these new products should get together with the regulators to get the products out in the field as quickly as possible. Next, he continued, "we need an evidence base for determining the most effective delivery and coverage to reach and then to sustain the public health goals that we aim for." This will require increased effort in implementation science. The National Institutes of Health now has a study section that funds implementation science, he said, but other groups should support it as well. Finally, Scott said, there is a growing consensus that no one approach will solve the problem by itself; combinations of interventions will be required. Thus, it will be important to build an evidence base concerning the effectiveness of various interventions, such as different types of vector control or vector-control programs combined with vaccines. However, carrying out phase 3 trials on various combinations of interventions would be logistically challenging and expensive. He suggested that there might be alternative ways to look at such combinations and decide which ones should move forward.

INTEGRATED SURVEILLANCE IN THE AMERICAS

Dos Santos began by noting that arboviruses have historically been a "high-visibility, high-priority topic" in the Americas. In 2003, PAHO adopted an integrated management strategy for dengue, and Zika and chikungunya were added in 2016. Unfortunately, that strategy has had little impact on transmission, dos Santos said. Part of the reason for the strategy's ineffectiveness is because so many of the drivers of transmission are outside of the health sector. However, he did note that there was a lull in transmission in the post-Zika years in 2017 and 2018, and then, as the

COVID-19 pandemic progressed and social distancing measures were put into place, there was a marked decrease in arboviral transmission in the latter part of 2020 and 2021.

For dengue alone, in 2023 up to the time of the workshop, there had been more than 4 million cases reported in the Americas through passive surveillance systems, dos Santos said, which was more annual cases of dengue since PAHO began keeping track in 1980. However, the case fatality rate remained below the regional target of 0.05 percent due to a targeted strategy of identifying "early predictors of severe disease at the primary health care setting," she said.

In the case of chikungunya, the year 2014—immediately after the virus's introduction into the Americas in 2013—recorded the largest number of cases by far (nearly 1.1 million), and in the several years following 2014 the total number of cases steadily dropped until it was less than 10 percent of that initial value. It has trended up somewhat since then, and Brazil, Paraguay, and other South American countries have experienced epidemics since 2022.

Concerning Zika, dos Santos said, there was an epidemic in 2016, but there has been relatively little activity since. "We are not seeing the sentinels, the canaries in the coal mine, if you will, of neurological disease clusters." It is difficult to get accurate data on the number of Zika cases because so many cases are asymptomatic or cause mild disease. For dengue, all four different serotypes have been circulating in the region, and the distribution of the serotypes has varied from country to country. In the first half of 2023, it was mostly dengue 1 and dengue 2 circulating, but in the second half of the year, dengue 3 and dengue 4 began playing a greater role in places like Guatemala, Costa Rica, and Mexico.

Next dos Santos spoke about collaborative surveillance and the Arbovirus Information Platform. The basic goal in implementing collaborative surveillance, she said, is to improve the amount and quality of evidence available for decision making. Granular data facilitates research and equips countries to guide their own interventions. To assemble that information, PAHO collects data from different streams, including case-based data, epidemiological surveillance data, entomological surveillance data, and laboratory data. PAHO transforms the country-provided data, unifying the data into a single format and depositing them into a single database. These transformed and aggregated arboviral surveillance data end up in two places. The first is PLISA, the Spanish acronym for the Health Information Platform for the Americas, which is publicly available.[2] The second is a collection of virtual collaboration spaces, which are private.

---

[2] PLISA can be accessed at https://opendata.paho.org/en.

The private collaboration spaces are "the mechanism through which we operationalize the collaborative surveillance," dos Santos said, and PAHO epidemiologists and systems engineers work with the country to tailor the virtual collaboration space to the country's needs and according to the data they have available. The potential for analysis depends on the number of variables collected by a country's surveillance strategy, she said, "but we try to tell the story that the data is trying to tell us in a compelling way." They use visualizations, charts, maps, and other techniques to make the data more useful, depending on what a country wants and needs, while still ensuring the security of the data. PAHO also has its own virtual collaboration space used to collaborate among the different areas of PAHO and the headquarters in Geneva. Some countries have agreements to share more granular data with each other through the virtual collaboration spaces than they make available publicly. There may be various details that the countries prefer not to be made public but that are important for neighboring countries to know so they can coordinate a multi-country response.

The virtual collaboration spaces offer a wealth of valuable information in various formats, such as epidemiological curves and maps, and in some countries the data are available at the subnational level. PAHO can provide special analyses, forecasts, and dashboards that allow officials in a country to get a clearer idea of what is happening in an outbreak or epidemic. When countries that have provided less information see the value that other countries are getting from the virtual collaboration spaces, she said, sometimes they will decide to start providing or collecting more data so that they can see the same benefit.

PAHO has been doing this for two years, working closely with the Centers for Disease Control and Prevention in Atlanta, during which time it has grown from 5 countries to 13. Speaking of lessons learned from this implementation, dos Santos noted the importance of trust, specifically that PAHO will not share or make data public unless a country authorizes it. A second lesson is that everyone should benefit. "This becomes sustainable when the country sees the benefit of this." If a country finds what PAHO offers to be useful, it will continue to take part. A third lesson is that integrated analysis catalyzes functional integration. "Putting those databases from case counts with entomological indicators drives an integrated response," she said, "because we are all looking at the same information, and we see our part in this map of telling the story of what's happening with these diseases." Fourth, PAHO has found its "come as you are" approach to be very useful. "We take the data however the country has it, in whatever format," dos Santos said. Working with existing data contributes to improved data quality and timeliness. Finally, PAHO started in the places with the highest likelihood of success to gain experience before moving on to areas where implementation could be more challenging.

Looking to the future, dos Santos said that PAHO is hoping to modernize and automate surveillance processes that are currently still manual and obsolete. PAHO will continue to use all available collected data—epidemiological, clinical, laboratory, entomological—to better understand transmission dynamics and apply prevention and control techniques most effectively. PAHO will also strengthen its capacities to improve data quality, analysis, integration, and decision making in prevention and control within national and subnational technical teams.

PREDICTIVE TOOLS AND MODELING

Brady, in the final presentation of the session, identified four different purposes for models: to better understand the process of arbovirus outbreaks, to improve the precision of estimates, to make predictions about the performance of different intervention options, and to forecast what will happen to a system in the future. He offered a general observation that modelers should use the simplest model that will answer their question and that sometimes the best approach is to create a model designed to answer a specific question rather than a very complicated one that can answer a collection of questions.

Models for Improving Understanding

Brady first looked at models of key epidemiological parameters for improving understanding and, specifically, for testing one hypothesis versus another concerning such things as immunity, climatic drivers, different aspects of the environment affecting the dynamics and transmission of viruses, or the origins of epidemics. This is often applied to hypotheses that are difficult to test experimentally, so data are retrospectively analyzed. As an example, he described how a model was used to understand why the Zika epidemic that hit the city of Salvador in northeast Brazil in 2015–2016 ended when it did. There was a big jump in cases, with the peak hitting around July 2015, and then an equally sharp drop-off (Netto et al., 2017). The two competing hypotheses for the epidemic ending was that the seasons changed and caused the weather to become unsuitable or that the population reached herd immunity.

Using seroprevalence data, Brady's group estimated the proportion of the population that had developed immunity, then fit and projected a model forward to 2016, assuming that the climate was similar to that of 2015. It predicted the epidemic would fizzle out because the percentage of the susceptible population had declined to a point where the epidemic could not continue, fitting what was subsequently seen in the real epidemic. The hypothesis that the epidemic ended because the population had reached herd immunity was supported.

Brady's group then took the understanding they got from that specific area in northeast Brazil to create a much more complicated model of 50 or so cities across Latin America to create projections of what would happen out to 2018. "We wouldn't have been able to do that if we didn't have a really clear understanding about what was driving the epidemic at a macro scale," he said. Modern models for understanding have gotten much more complex, Brady said, specifically for dengue. A study analyzing dengue emergence in Vietnam found that while heavy rain and drought lead to more dengue, this relationship weakens in areas with higher provision of piped water, suggesting expanding access to piped water may protect against extreme weather events (Gibb et al., 2023).

Several factors have made such detailed models possible, Brady said. The biggest factor has been the rapidly growing amounts of publicly available data on disease cases that are presented at higher spatial and temporal resolutions. There are also many more datasets available on explanatory variables such as infrastructure, human movement, and climate and other environment variables. In the future, he predicted, the models will be improved by including causal inference methods, which should provide more of a theoretical basis to the models and perhaps lead to a more consistent understanding of the drivers of transmission.

Models for Estimation

Models for estimation can increase precision concerning specific parameters that are useful for arbovirus control, such as reproduction number, burden, and effectiveness. "Models can fill the gap where experimental measurement is impractical or impossible," Brady said. For example, reproduction number, the average number of new infections generated by a single infected individual, is a key factor in determining whether an outbreak is growing or contracting. However, it is a very difficult number to measure directly, particularly for vector-borne diseases, because chains of transmission cannot be directly observed, so it must be inferred from case data. Burden must also be estimated with models. It is impractical to measure disease burden globally because there are too many data gaps. As a result, many of the disease burden figures that are given for dengue, yellow fever, chikungunya, and Zika are model-based estimates.

Models are also used for estimating the efficacy of interventions in a trial. For things like vector control, an intervention will apply to an area rather than individuals, so it is not possible to do a randomized, controlled trial on individuals; it is instead necessary to work with clusters, and generally there will be some level of contamination between the control and intervention clusters. Modeling makes it possible to get around this constraint, Brady said. "If we have a good idea about how much movement of mosquitoes, of people, of transmission coupling there is between these areas, we can take the results of the trial and remove that contamination to get a more precise estimate of what the true efficacy is."

Concerning future developments related to using modeling for estimation, Brady shared that a key step will be expanding to other disciplines, such as measuring the effectiveness of vector-control programs. He also suggested that modeling could be used to inform trial design and that it would be useful to target data collection to improve modeled estimates.

Models for Prediction

Brady explained that modeling for prediction is scenario-based. It is about predicting the consequences of different intervention choices, such as figuring out the best long-term strategy for a new intervention or how best to combine multiple interventions together at a scale that cannot be measured experimentally. Being able to predict the consequences of interventions is increasingly critical for obtaining investment in new types of interventions. An example of this was the Sanofi Pasteur dengue modeling comparison group, which had seven different modeling teams predicting effectiveness across different settings (Flasche et al., 2016). It is very important, Brady said, to have multiple modeling groups with different assumptions and different interpretations of the data involved in these big decisions. In another case, a team led by Brady looked at how the cost-effectiveness of using *Wolbachia* would vary spatially (Brady et al., 2020). The modeling showed that the intervention is most cost-effective in high-density, high-burden cities, and now *Wolbachia* interventions often prioritize such cities. A third example is using modeling to predict the effects of combining interventions, which is generally not practical to study in trials. One recent study modeled the effects of combining dengue control programs in the state of Yucatán, Mexico (Hladish et al., 2020).

The enabling factors for model predictions have been good collaborations with intervention developers, governments, and international health organizations along with more work between modelers to build consensus on the models. Future developments will include more realistic and locally relevant predictions, which should improve robustness.

Models for Forecasting

The idea underlying the use of models for forecasting is fairly simple, Brady said. "For vector-borne diseases, there's a lag between the climate you observe and the outcome that you [later] observe with dengue cases. Rainfall leads to high [numbers of] mosquito[es] leads to infection, and there's a 2-week to 1-month gap between those." Thus, vector-borne diseases are more amenable to forecasting than some other diseases. The Dengue Forecasting Model Satellite-Based System (D-MOSS) for Vietnam is a particularly advanced model that includes a super-ensemble of 50 different models he said (Colón-González et al., 2021). The Vietnamese government uses it to decide how to respond to epidemics. It has also expanded to Malaysia and is starting to be used in Sri Lanka. The model's short-term forecasts are useful for immediate control, such as spraying of insecticides. Medium-term forecasts help public health officials plan for the coming months, and long-term forecasts inform such decisions as the size of the budget that will be needed in the coming year.

In summary, Brady shared that a growing understanding of the drivers of arboviruses, more efficient Bayesian inference methods, and more relevant approaches to validation developed with ministries of health have enabled the development of more advanced models. Co-development with ministries of health, he continued, has also been instrumental in identifying the facets of disease outbreaks that need to be predicted. In the future Brady would like to see more evaluation of forecasts. "We want to do a clustered, randomized, controlled trial to show [whether] forecasting actually has an impact." Concluding, Brady said that the development of models is not just about building better models but also is about working better with other groups so that modeling is used in practical situations to help with the control of and response to arbovirus outbreaks.

DISCUSSION

In response to a question as to whether PAHO might take unilateral action based on data from its monitoring network, dos Santos first noted that since PAHO is monitoring the data with the countries, the organization generally does not see things a country has not seen. However, she said, sometimes PAHO might notice a pattern across countries, such as more and more countries crossing their epidemic thresholds, at which point PAHO issues an "epi-alert," which warns countries that they are anticipating an intense season for arboviral disease. PAHO issued six epi-alerts for arboviral diseases in 2023 alone, she said, but PAHO does not act in opposition to a country's wishes.

Next, Scott was asked a question about how climate change may be affecting populations of vectors such as mosquitoes and ticks. Scott said that weather certainly affects vector populations, but connections to climate change are less clear. For example, Scott noted that laboratory research has shown that temperature fluctuations affect how viruses interact with the vectors. Scott also mentioned a study he was involved in that concluded that climate change could affect the distribution of mosquitoes, although not necessarily their overall abundance "because in some places they would go away, and in other places they would show up."

Climate change is important, Gubler commented, and it influences arboviral diseases, but the current focus on the effects of climate change on arboviral disease are misleading and taking away attention from other important issues. For instance, increased flooding is one effect associated with climate change, but in the case of most arboviruses, flooding decreases transmission instead of increasing it, "because it floods all of the larval habitats away, and it takes weeks to sometimes months for those mosquito populations to come back." Furthermore, he continued, the focus on climate change can take money away from public health projects and research on vector-borne diseases, which instead goes to climate change research.

A participant asked Scott about indoor residual sprays leading to pesticide resistance in the mosquitoes, noting that residual spraying had not worked well in Singapore because of such resistance. It is a major problem, Scott acknowledged, but strategies such as targeted indoor residual spraying cuts down the amount of insecticide that is delivered and the amount of time it takes to deliver it. Lenhart expanded on that by discussing a large clustered, randomized trial in Mexico that is monitoring for insecticide resistance. After 2 years of targeted application, mosquitoes have retained susceptibility. Although the emergence of resistance is always going to be a risk when an insecticide is being used, Lenhart said, the approach being used in the trial is a "much more logical way of applying the insecticide" than typical schemes.

Paz-Bailey then offered a comment about new vector-control strategies. In particular, she pointed to the use of *Wolbachia* replacement methods, in which large numbers of *Aedes* mosquitoes infected with *Wolbachia* bacteria are released into an area to compete with and interact with the other mosquitoes there. Studies have shown that it greatly reduces the rates of transmission of such arboviruses as dengue, Zika, and chikungunya, and Paz-Bailey indicated that "in the field, *Wolbachia* replacement seems to show a lot of hope."

Next, a question was posed about the need for a national or international clearinghouse structure among federal agencies and countries that could announce the detection of certain invasive species that may spread disease and could help speed up detection and response. Scott answered that effective detection efforts for *Aedes*-borne viruses must start at the local level, but ultimately "you would want to have something that was structured across countries within a region." Brady added that such a system does exist in the European Union, and it has been important for tracking arbovirus vectors through France, Germany, and the UK. However, he added, it is only useful in Western Europe because of large gaps in surveillance in Eastern Europe.

The session's final question concerned the types of data that will be needed to get insight into the complex interactions that affect vaccine success. Dos Santos answered that more information is needed about what interventions are being done, where they are located, and the vaccine status of people living in the areas of interest. Brady added that the "ability to pick apart interactions is really boosted by the amount of follow-up," even if just from regular collection of case data. Serological data are also important, he added.

Scott then spoke about the interactions between vaccine and vector control. Vaccines elevate herd immunity, and vector control lowers the force of infection. "The vaccine would make vector control sustainable." However, experience in Singapore has shown that it is possible to have very low numbers of mosquitoes and still have an outbreak if herd immunity is low enough, he added. "So, the real question here is what sort of protection from infection do the vaccines give?" Scott continued. "If the vaccines don't protect against infection, then this whole scenario doesn't work."

REFERENCES

Brady, O. J., D. D. Kharisma, N. N. Wilastonegoro, K. M. O'Reilly, E. Hendrickx, L. S. Bastos, L. Yakob, and D. S. Shepard. 2020. The cost-effectiveness of controlling dengue in Indonesia using wMel *Wolbachia* released at scale: A modelling study. *BMC Medicine* 18(1):186.

Colón-González, F. J., L. Soares Bastos, B. Hofmann, A. Hopkin, Q. Harpham, T. Crocker, R. Amato, I. Ferrario, F. Moschini, S. James, S. Malde, E. Ainscoe, V. Sinh Nam, D. Quang Tan, N. Duc Khoa, M. Harrison, G. Tsarouchi, D. Lumbroso, O. J. Brady, and R. Lowe. 2021. Probabilistic seasonal dengue forecasting in Vietnam: A modelling study using superensembles. *PLOS Medicine* 18(3):e1003542.

Dadzie, S. K., J. Akorli, M. B. Coulibaly, K. M. Ahadji-Dabla, I. Baber, T. Bobanga, A. O. M. S. Boukhary, T. Canelas, L. Facchinelli, A. Gonçalves, M. Guelbeogo, B. Kamgang, I. K. Keita, L. Konan, R. Levine, N. Dzuris, A. Lenhart, and WAASuN contributors. 2022. Building the capacity of West African countries in *Aedes* surveillance: Inaugural meeting of the West African Aedes Surveillance Network (WAASuN). *Parasites & Vectors* 15(1):381.

Eisen, L. 2020. Stemming the rising tide of human-biting ticks and tickborne diseases, United States. *Emerging Infectious Diseases* 26(4):641–647.

Flasche, S., M. Jit, I. Rodríguez-Barraquer, L. Coudeville, M. Recker, K. Koelle, G. Milne, T. J. Hladish, T. A. Perkins, D. A. Cummings, I. Dorigatti, D. J. Laydon, G. España, J. Kelso, I. Longini, J. Lourenco, C. A. Pearson, R. C. Reiner, L. Mier-Y-Terán-Romero, K. Vannice, and N. Ferguson. 2016. The long-term safety, public health impact, and cost-effectiveness of routine vaccination with a recombinant, live-attenuated dengue vaccine (Dengvaxia): A model comparison study. *PLOS Medicine* 13(11):e1002181.

Gibb, R., F. J. Colón-González, P. T. Lan, P. T. Huong, V. S. Nam, V. T. Duoc, D. T. Hung, N. T. Dong, V. C. Chien, L. T. T. Trang, D. Kien Quoc, T. M. Hoa, N. H. Tai, T. T. Hang, G. Tsarouchi, E. Ainscoe, Q. Harpham, B. Hofmann, D. Lumbroso, O. J. Brady, and R. Lowe. 2023. Interactions between climate change, urban infrastructure, and mobility are driving dengue emergence in Vietnam. *Nature Communications* 14(1):8179.

Hladish, T. J., C. A. B. Pearson, K. B. Toh, D. P. Rojas, P. Manrique-Saide, G. M. Vazquez-Prokopec, M. E. Halloran, and I. M. Longini Jr. 2020. Designing effective control of dengue with combined interventions. *Proceedings of the National Academies of Sciences* 117(6):3319–3325.

Keesing, F., S. Mowry, W. Bremer, S. Duerr, A. S. Evans Jr., I. R. Fischhoff, A. F. Hinckley, S. A. Hook, F. Keating, J. Pendleton, A. Pfister, M. Teator, and R. S. Ostfeld. 2022. Effects of tick-control interventions on tick abundance, human encounters with ticks, and incidence of tickborne diseases in residential neighborhoods, New York, USA. *Emerging Infectious Diseases* 28(5):957–966.

Montalvo Zurbia-Flores, G., C. S. Rollier, and A. Reyes-Sandoval. 2022. Re-thinking yellow fever vaccines: Fighting old foes with new generation vaccines. *Human Vaccines & Immunotherapeutics* 18(1):1895644.

Netto, E. M., A. Moreira-Soto. C. Pedroso, C. Höser, S. Funk, A. J. Kucharski, A. Rockstroh, B. M. Kümmerer, G. S. Sampaio, E. Luz, S. N. Vaz, J. P. Dias F. A. Bastos, R. Cabral, T. Kistemann, S. Ulbert, X. de Lamballerie, T. Jaenisch, O. J. Brady, C. Drosten, M. Sarno, C. Brites, and J. F. Drexler. 2017. High Zika virus seroprevalence in Salvador, northeastern Brazil limits the potential for further outbreaks. *mBio* 8:6.

Roiz, D., A. L. Wilson, T. W. Scott, D. M. Fonseca, F. Jourdain, P. Müller, R. Velayudhan, and V. Corbel. 2018. Integrated *Aedes* management for the control of *Aedes*-borne diseases. *PLOS Neglected Tropical Diseases* 12(12):e0006845.

Stafford, K. C. 2004. *Tick Management Handbook: An Integrated Guide for Homeowners, Pest Control Operators, and Public Health Officials for the Prevention of Tick-Associated Disease.* Atlanta, GA: Centers for Disease Control and Prevention.

Vannice, K. S., S. L. Hills, L. M. Schwartz, A. D. Barrett, J. Heffelfinger, J. Hombach, G. W. Letson, T. Solomon, A. A. Marfin, and the Japanese Encephalitis Vaccination Experts Panel. 2021. The future of Japanese encephalitis vaccination: Expert recommendations for achieving and maintaining optimal JE control. *npj Vaccines* 6(1):82.

Wilson, A. L., M. Boelaert, I. Kleinschmidt, M. Pinder, T. W. Scott, L. S. Tusting, and S. W. Lindsay. 2015. Evidence-based vector control? Improving the quality of vector control trials. *Trends in Parasitology* 31(8):380–390.

WHO (World Health Organization). 2017. *How to design vector control efficacy trials: Guidance on phase III vector control field trial design provided by the Vector Control Advisory Group.* Geneva, Switzerland: World Health Organization. https://policycommons.net/artifacts/545768/how-to-design-vector-control-efficacy-trials/1523325/ (accessed February 1, 2024).

5

Lessons Learned from Previous Outbreaks

Highlights

- It is vital to maintain diagnostic capacity to be ready to deal with outbreaks as soon as they occur instead of having to take time to build up that capacity. (Staples)
- Maintaining an awareness and surveillance infrastructure is important for arbovirus detection, monitoring, and control efforts. Challenges in the United States include a decline in the number of state entomologists over the years. (Staples)
- It is crucial to continue to work on knowledge gaps in between outbreaks to be more prepared to deal with future ones. (Staples)
- New approaches to regulation are needed for dealing with outbreaks, as the current regulatory approach significantly increases response times. (Staples)
- Various drivers will push the emergence of viral and arbovirus infections in the coming years, including urbanization, deforestation, animal and human migrations, poverty, political instability, and climate change. (Hotez)
- Chronic noncommunicable diseases such as diabetes and hypertension will play a role in future arbovirus outbreaks. (Hotez)
- Fragmentation in health care systems will limit the effectiveness of response to future arbovirus outbreaks. (Hotez)

continued

- It is important to pay attention to vaccines and other technologies that can be developed and used locally in low- and middle-income countries. (Hotez)
- Anti-vaccine and anti-science attitudes in the public will make it more difficult to deploy some of the advanced vaccines and technologies being developed to address arbovirus diseases. (Hotez)

NOTE: These points were made by the individual workshop speakers/participants identified above. They are not intended to reflect a consensus among workshop participants.

Each viral outbreak can offer an opportunity to learn how to respond better to future outbreaks. As forum vice chair and session moderator Kent E. Kester explained, the workshop's fourth session was devoted to hearing about lessons that have been learned from previous outbreaks in order to help shape preparedness and response efforts for future arboviral outbreaks.

The session panel had two speakers. The first was Erin Staples, a medical epidemiologist in the Arboviral Diseases Branch of the Centers for Disease Control and Prevention (CDC), who spoke about lessons learned from previous arboviral outbreaks. The second was Peter Hotez, the dean of the National School of Tropical Medicine and a professor of pediatrics and molecular virology at the Baylor College of Medicine in Houston. Hotez spoke about lessons from dealing with the COVID-19 pandemic that can be applied to arboviruses. A question-and-answer period followed their presentations.

PREVIOUS ARBOVIRAL OUTBREAKS

Staples began by listing more than two dozen arboviral outbreaks and emergence events from the past 20 years. There were multiple outbreaks of chikungunya, West Nile virus, yellow fever, and Zika as well as so many dengue outbreaks that she did not even list them individually. Less common outbreaks and emergence events included eastern equine encephalitis, western equine encephalitis, Japanese encephalitis, Bourbon virus, Heartland virus, and severe fever with thrombocytopenia syndrome. Staples was involved in the response to more than a dozen of those, she said, and her talk focused on four specific lessons she learned from those experiences.

The first lesson was the importance of ensuring diagnostic capacity. There is always normal seasonal variation in the number of diagnostic samples the CDC receives at its Arboviral Diseases Laboratory, but when an outbreak begins, the numbers can dramatically increase. The 2014 chikungunya outbreak in the Americas, for instance, led to a threefold increase in the number of samples the CDC received; the agency was able to handle that jump in testing with relative ease because it had prepared reagents ahead of time that it could send out to state health departments and increase testing capacity. A more severe challenge came with the 2016 Zika outbreak, Staples said, when "all of a sudden, instead of getting 150 samples a month to test with our limited staff, we had over 4,000 samples pouring into our laboratory" (Figure 5-1). That forced the agency to call in additional resources. "Our bacterial diseases lab became an arboviral lab," she said. "The Atlanta labs became arboviral labs." But again, because of the stocks of reagents and the ability to bring in extra testing capacity, the CDC was able to respond to the surge in demand.

These experiences showed, Staples said, the importance of maintaining a surge capacity for arboviral disease testing; that surge capacity depends on having adequate stores of reagents and control materials, establishing sample-sharing policies, and maintaining common testing platforms. One issue that needs to be addressed, Staples said, is the role of laboratory-developed tests in a public health response. If a new arbovirus appears for which there are no existing tests, laboratory-developed tests will be important in the response. However, she added that regulatory requirements would pose an additional obstacle in a public health response.

A second lesson, Staples said, is the importance of maintaining global awareness for arboviral diseases as well as the infrastructure necessary to

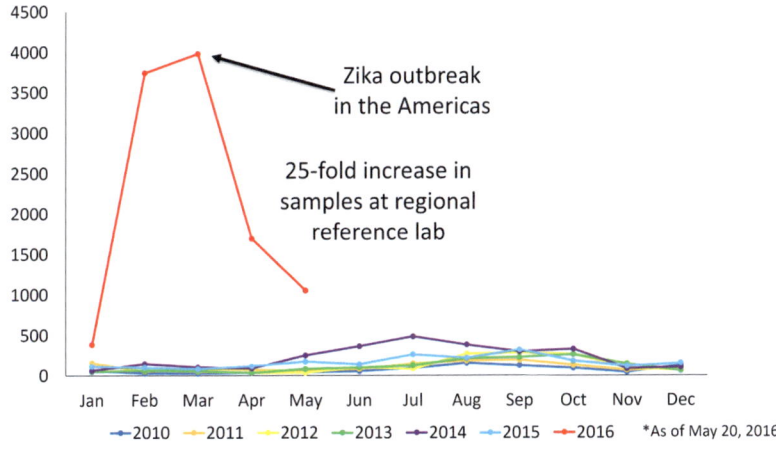

FIGURE 5-1 Number of diagnostic samples received at the CDC's Arboviral Diseases Branch diagnostics laboratory by month from January 2010 to May 2016.
SOURCES: Presented by Erin Staples on December 12, 2023; CDC, 2023.

monitor them. As an example, she pointed to the experience with Zika. The measured numbers of Zika cases peaked in 2016, but the numbers of cases of microcephaly associated with the Zika virus peaked in late 2015 or early 2016, and the infections leading to those cases would have occurred in 2015. Thus, she said, "we probably had just as many if not more infections in 2015 due to Zika virus, but we just didn't know about it. We weren't aware, we weren't looking for it."

One current stumbling block to maintaining awareness for arboviral diseases in the United States, Staples suggested, is the lack of emphasis placed on such awareness by the states. In 1927, every state had a state entomologist because of efforts to eradicate malaria, but in 2022 there were only 16 state entomologists. Similarly, in 2022 there was very spotty surveillance and reporting of the West Nile virus in mosquitoes—and the areas without state entomologists were much less likely to be carrying out such surveillance. "Awareness and surveillance infrastructures are very important for detecting and monitoring and control efforts," she said, and the United States does not have a comprehensive system of monitoring for nonhuman disease vectors.

In short, Staples concluded, maintaining surveillance infrastructure is important for detection, monitoring, and control efforts and could be accomplished by maintaining arboviral expertise at the state level. Optimally, arboviral surveillance could include human, vector, and animal components, as applicable. For instance, observing deaths in nonhuman primates can provide a warning signal of an impending outbreak of yellow fever in South America. Unfortunately, she continued, most areas of the world lack adequate vector surveillance. Furthermore, the integration of animal data with other surveillance data is a significant challenge.

The third lesson, Staples said, is that it is important to continue to address knowledge gaps. As an example, she showed a graph of the last 50 years of Zika virus publications. There were very few for most of that time, then the numbers grew quickly after the outbreak and peaked at about 2,000 publications during the year after the outbreak but then dropped sharply; in 2023 there were only half the number of publications as in 2016. Furthermore, the number of publications on Zika in 2023 were just a little more than 1 percent of the number of publications on coronavirus. In short, she said, "we haven't done a great job . . . of addressing the gaps that remained at the end of the [Zika] outbreak."

Continuing, Staples identified five specific knowledge gaps that remain after the Zika outbreak in the Americas. First is the potential for nonhuman circulation of the virus and its endemicity. Second is the identification of the optimal diagnostic testing for congenital Zika virus syndrome. Another knowledge gap exists around potential antibody-dependent enhancement of Zika virus infections with dengue virus infections. Fourth, if a vaccine is developed, which epitopes are most important for vaccine neutralization, and what can be done to decrease the cross-reactivity that could occur? Finally, what can be learned about time intervals between outbreaks and when should the system be prepared for the next outbreak? "I don't have an answer for that right now," she said.

Addressing these knowledge gaps is complicated by a lack of sustained funding and competing public health priorities, Staples said. "We just don't have adequate resources." In the future, it may be important to have existing protocols and networks readily available to address the knowledge gaps. Staples illustrated that "by the time we implemented the network for pregnant women to look at the impacts of Zika, the outbreak was almost over, and we weren't able to generate enough data." So, protocols should be established prior to outbreaks to allow them to be quickly implemented as part of the response efforts. She also noted that improving partnerships among industry, academia, and government will be an important step in overcoming these challenges and effectively addressing the gaps in knowledge about Zika and other arboviral diseases.

The fourth lesson that Staples offered was the importance of considering alternative agreements and regulatory needs. A response to an arboviral outbreak requires many different components, such as surveillance, laboratory testing, vector control, medical countermeasures, and community engagement, and each of these components requires its own infrastructure. But there are various hurdles that arise in these different areas that can slow a response, particularly hurdles related to regulatory approval pathways. Product approval is an area where slowdowns can occur, but there are many others, such as the need for approval from an institutional review board for testing on human subjects or resistance to the use of insecticides. "All of those things take time," Staples said. "The existing mechanisms really are not great, and because we always hit those roadblocks, we need to think about how to overcome some of these issues that we face." Increasing regulatory requirements are there for a good reason, she said, but they are affecting readiness and may need to be modified in the case of urgent public health responses.

In closing, Staples offered some suggestions for how to be prepared to respond to the next arboviral disease outbreak. First, she said, "We have to expect the unexpected. We didn't expect Zika virus was going to cause microcephaly." Second, it will be important to define likely hotspots for emergence and target them for surveillance. Third, regulatory pathways should be developed for preapproving common arboviral test platforms such as the enzyme-linked immunosorbent assay (ELISA), so that they can be put to work quickly in an outbreak. "If we had approval of these test platforms, we could swap out our antigens, we could swap out our reagents, and we could be more versatile to potentially have early detection but also early response," she said. Fourth, it is important to foster more open regulatory discussions for countermeasures to allow obstacles to be addressed proactively.

Staples noted that another important step will be to advance considerations for alternative mosquito control techniques against multiple mosquito species. No single technique is going to work against all the types of mosquitoes, she said. Finally, she concluded, there needs to be increased coordination between public and private entities and their overlapping efforts. Different entities have developed dengue vaccines that are most effective against different strains, Staples said. It would make sense to combine the work to find a marker that would provide effective cross-protective immunity against all strains, she said. "We need to work together."

COVID-19

Hotez began by saying that although he is not an arbovirologist, he has learned about arboviruses by working on the Gulf Coast for the past 12 years and going through Zika and dengue outbreaks. His remarks centered around five lessons learned from working with COVID-19 that could be applied to dealing with arboviruses.

The first lesson, Hotez said, is that there are a number of key twenty-first century drivers leading to the emergence of viral infections, including arbovirus infections. In his book *Preventing the Next Pandemic: Vaccine Diplomacy in a Time of Anti-Science* (2021), Hotez examined how poverty, war, political instability, urbanization, deforestation, human and animal migrations, and climate change are combining in unique and interesting ways to increase the risk of pandemics. For instance, as more of the world's population is moving to urban areas, a new generation of megacities is appearing in higher-, middle-, and lower-income countries simultaneously. Unfortunately, many of these megacities are sweltering, with their average temperatures being steadily increased by global warning, which creates more hospitable environments for *Aedes* mosquitoes, especially *Aedes aegypti*. The widespread poverty that is found in many of these megacities also plays a role in the risk of arbovirus emergence and spread, as does political instability and increasing deforestation.

Many of the world's hotspots where sharp increases in disease can be observed—places like the Arabian Peninsula, parts of Africa, parts of central Latin America, and Texas and the Gulf Coast—are places where there is a combination of urbanization, climate change and deforestation, political instability, and other twenty-first century forces. A good illustration of these forces in practice, Hotez said, is what has been happening on the Arabian Peninsula since the 2010s. The ISIS occupation of parts of Syria and Iraq and the civil war in Yemen forced people to crowd into cities, and then an explosion in sand fly populations led to hyper-endemic leishmaniasis. There were also dengue outbreaks. Unprecedented temperatures of 50°C or more forced people to abandon agricultural pursuits along the Tigris and Euphrates rivers and flee into Aleppo and Damascus, which fueled exposure to vectors and vector-borne illnesses, and the situation was exacerbated by a halting of vaccination programs. "So, the Middle East was a good crucible of all of those forces together," Hotez said, "and you had the largest cholera outbreak that the world had seen in some time in Yemen because of that."

Something similar happened in central Latin America following the socioeconomic collapse of the Maduro regime in Venezuela. Vector-control programs and immunization programs were discontinued, and unemployed people sought employment in the illegal gold mining industry and ended up sleeping outdoors without mosquito nets. "So, you saw this massive rise in malaria cases as well as dengue and others," Hotez said. And even along the American Gulf Coast there are predictions that warming temperatures will lead to rising numbers of *Aedes* mosquitoes and then to increasing numbers of cases of dengue, chikungunya, and Zika virus infections (Hotez et al., 2014).

Unfortunately, he continued, there has been little attention paid to the looming risk of arboviruses in that area, so he and a colleague published an article in the *New England Journal of Medicine* calling attention to the vulnerability to these diseases along the Gulf Coast (Hotez and LaBeaud, 2023). "I think this discussion is important to elevate arboviruses to the same attention of the policy makers that they have for some of the catastrophic respiratory illnesses," he said.

The risk along the Gulf Coast is due to a combination of factors—not just climate change but also human migration, aggressive urbanization, and poverty. The reason poverty is so important, Hotez explained, is that poorer people are more likely to live in dilapidated homes with no window screens and an absence of air conditioning, which means they keep their windows open when it is hot. This is combined with the fact that many people in low-income neighborhoods dump their tires, which hold water and serve as breeding grounds for mosquitoes. "We do have *Aedes aegypti* mosquitoes here in Houston," he said, "and that's important."

As an aside, Hotez noted that he has been working with Senator Cory Booker (Dem.-NJ) on legislation called STOP: Study, Treat, Observe and Prevent Neglected Diseases,[1] which is designed to raise awareness of the importance of doing better surveillance for arboviruses and neglected tropical diseases on the Gulf Coast and in the southern United States.

---

[1] *STOP Neglected Diseases of Poverty Act*, S. 324, 118th Congress, 1st sess., Congressional Record 169, no. 27, daily ed. (February 9, 2023).

A second lesson to be learned from COVID-19, Hotez said, is the role played by chronic underlying noncommunicable diseases, such as diabetes and cardiovascular diseases. The rates of these diseases are climbing not only in the United States but also globally. Diabetes is hitting both the African continent and India very hard, for instance. The COVID-19 pandemic showed how important diabetes and hypertension were as risk factors for that disease, but the literature shows that they are also important risk factors for dengue (Mehta and Hotez, 2016).

Conversely, the viruses themselves have chronic and persistent effects. The existence of long COVID is well known, but influenza and other viruses produce long-term, chronic, and debilitating effects as well. This has been demonstrated for West Nile virus, he said, and it may be true for other arboviruses as well (Garcia et al., 2015).

A third factor shown to be important with COVID-19, and likely to be important for arboviral diseases, is the fragmentation of the country's health systems, Hotez said, especially for arbovirus control. "Here in Harris County and Houston, Texas, we have two health departments, both the city and the county, and a very well-run mosquito control division," he said. "They do surveillance, they're doing PCR (polymerase chain reaction), they're monitoring for viruses." But the problem, he continued, is that other Texas counties, particularly some of the more rural or less wealthy counties, do not have such well-run monitoring and control programs. Addressing the variability between counties in terms of mosquito and virus surveillance and control is going to be very important, he said.

A fourth lesson is the importance of remembering the needs of lower- and middle-income countries when developing vaccines and other technologies to deal with arboviruses. In the case of COVID-19, Hotez said, in 2021 much of the African continent and the Indian subcontinent lagged far behind the rest of the world in vaccination rates, "in part because there was so much emphasis on speed and innovation and cool technologies like messenger RNA (mRNA) and particle vaccines." Perhaps vaccine distribution may have been more globally equitable if older technologies had been available to manufacture locally.

To address this issue, a group of vaccine producers in low- and middle-income countries organized the Developing Country Vaccine Manufacturers Network and have developed and provided vaccines for such diseases as hepatitis B (Hayman and Pagliusi, 2020). "The point is, yes, we want cutting edge technologies but also to figure out a way to be compatible with the vaccine producers in the low- and middle-income countries," Hotez said. "You don't have to be a big pharma company to still do big things, and looking at models that go beyond the big pharma companies could be extremely helpful."

Finally, Hotez said, "I think we should not underestimate the impact of the anti-vaccine movement." Some 200,000 Americans needlessly died because they refused the COVID-19 vaccine, he said, and the anti-vaccine movement is not stopping at COVID-19 but extending into childhood immunizations as well (Hotez, 2023). Furthermore, it is globalizing. It has moved into Canada and Europe and even Latin America. Although there are exciting new vaccines becoming available for arboviruses, such as a chikungunya vaccine and a couple of dengue vaccines, it is not clear how well they will be accepted. A particular concern is the yellow fever vaccine, which has rare but serious side effects. Additionally, the anti-science movement does not threaten only vaccines. Such interventions as the *Wolbachia* bacteria and genetically modified mosquitoes may also meet resistance. "I think there's going to be a big barrier that we are not really addressing," Hotez said.

Summarizing, Hotez said that he believes there is an arbovirus tsunami coming, and the public health field is not ready. "We are not ready because of this new paradigm of hot and sweltering megacities with climate change, urbanization, urban poverty. We are not ready because of the unprecedented levels of diabetes and hypertension which is going to increase the severity of arbovirus infections. We still have a fragmented health system." Furthermore, he concluded, not enough attention is being paid to accelerating technologies locally in low- and middle-income countries or to the way that anti-science could slow the uptake of new vector control technologies, vaccines, medicines, and diagnostics.

DISCUSSION

Rebecca Gustafson from Louisiana State University began the discussion session with a question about raising awareness concerning the risks that poor populations face from arboviral diseases as well as the elevated risks that arise in the wake of various disasters, such as hurricanes. Hotez responded by noting that the poor are more susceptible to the effects of catastrophic weather events because they tend to live in weather- and climate-vulnerable areas where people with means do not want to live, such as the low-lying areas around New Orleans that were most affected by Hurricane Katrina. Second, people living in low-income neighborhoods are likely to be more susceptible to mosquito-borne illnesses because there are likely to be more places for mosquitoes to breed, such as in discarded tires for *Aedes aegypti* mosquitoes or drainage ditches for *Culex* mosquitoes. A third factor, Hotez said, is that many policy makers do not understand that disease transmission occurs in the United States. One of the reasons Hotez cited as why he started working with Senator Booker is to raise awareness of the risks created by the combination of warming temperatures, altered rainfall patterns, urbanization, and extreme poverty. But, he continued, getting those messages out has been "extremely tough and challenging."

Kester then asked both panelists what it would take to increase public and private investment in the prevention of arboviral disease. Staples said that one approach is to talk about it in cost–benefit terms—for instance, what 5 million cases of dengue a year cost society and what it would cost to take some simple preventive measures. "A can of spray foam to plug up holes in a tree [to control La Crosse virus vectors] is $10," she said. "You could buy a lot of spray foam and prevent a lot of disease burden and costs in a very simple way."

Hotez agreed and added that both the United States and the G20 countries have committed to funding programs for pandemic preparedness. The problem, though, is that people are thinking mainly about respiratory viruses like SARS-CoV-2 or sometimes the filoviruses, such as Ebola, which cause severe hemorrhagic fever. "The key is getting a seat at the table for the arboviruses, getting people to understand that these are every bit as important and every bit a threat as anything else," he said, "and recognize there are some unique aspects for arboviruses that would not be covered in general use funds for respiratory viruses."

Kester then asked Hotez to comment on the current push to develop mRNA vaccines in the wake of their success against COVID-19, particularly since there is no guarantee that they will be as successful against other types of diseases. "I think everyone is running to the mRNA basket, and I think that's a mistake," Hotez replied. While mRNA is certainly a promising technology, he said, it is not necessarily the best technology for vaccines against all the different pathogens. More importantly, it is wise to have multiple options for when a new epidemic occurs because it is never clear in advance which will prove to be the most effective for the disease and context of the outbreak. "We should be getting as many technologies in play as possible" to prepare for future arbovirus outbreaks, he said.

Another problem to consider, Hotez said, is how to make sure that low- and middle-income countries can quickly access the vaccines they need in an outbreak. One approach is simply building up the vaccine-manufacturing infrastructure and capacity in those countries. Another issue that needs to be addressed is regulation. "We had this problem where everything had to go through the WHO [World Health Organization] prequalification mechanism, and they wound up sitting on a lot of technologies coming out of the developing country vaccine producers and putting a velvet rope around the big pharma companies." As a result, low- and middle-income countries ended up relying on vaccine makers in the United States, Europe, and Japan and had to wait in line.

In response to another question, Hotez suggested that the current focus on climate change could be used to help get more attention paid to arbovirus prevention. "Let's make the case that the reason why arboviruses have to have a seat at the pandemic preparedness table is because these are the viruses of climate change."

Responding to a comment about the lack of interest in developing a Zika vaccine once the Zika outbreak was contained, Hotez suggested that it might make sense to move toward developing a pan-arbovirus vaccine that would be effective against many different viruses. For instance, he continued, when the drug representatives for Merck speak about their tetravalent dengue vaccine, which can handle all four versions of dengue, he wonders, "why aren't we making this a pentavalent vaccine and adding a component for Zika, or a hexavalent vaccine and adding in chikungunya, or even heptavalent with West Nile?" Currently people are not thinking in those terms, he said, but there should be an effort to "lift all boats simultaneously" by targeting not only dengue for vaccination but also other arboviruses.

Following a question about equity, both Staples and Hotez agreed that it will be important to work for greater equity in the prevention and control of arboviruses, but they also agreed that it is a challenging issue. "I think we need to advocate . . . in general for arboviruses," Staples said, "because no matter where you go in the world, other than maybe Antarctica, you will have an arbovirus that is going to be impacting someone. . . . Talk globally, and advocate for all of our viruses together because that way we are going to make sure we engage the right people."

Hotez agreed, saying that the equity lens can be powerful, but it is not easy to work with. He spoke of a time after he had a great success working with the U.S. Congress on packages of mass treatment for neglected tropical diseases such as intestinal worms, schistosomiasis, and river blindness, and then he returned to the same people to talk about neglected tropical diseases in the United States, including arboviruses. Hotez said that their response was "Yeah, Peter, but before you were talking about a simple package of pills. Now you're telling us we have to go into infected communities, we've got to do surveillance, there are issues around quality housing, doing cleanup of low-income neighborhoods, preventive measures. This is messy, Peter." So, he concluded, moving forward on measures to prevent arboviruses can be a tough sell.

One participant asked the panelists to comment on the role that health care systems play in the effort to protect against arboviruses. Hotez described a study by Murray et al. (2013) looking at patients presenting to Houston area hospitals in 2003–2005, which found that there had been a cluster of dengue cases coming into Houston-area emergency rooms—and probably locally transmitted dengue between 2003 and 2005—but that almost none of those cases, including one that resulted in death, were diagnosed at the time. Part of the reason, he said, is that health care professionals in the United States do not think about such illnesses as dengue. The lesson, he said, is "we have to do a better job of raising awareness [about arboviral diseases] among the doctors, the nurses, and health care professionals, particularly as we head into summer and fall months. . . . People just don't think about these conditions."

Staples said that such education will need to be tailored according to where in the world doctors, nurses, and other health care professionals are practicing. "When I've been in Africa, it's malaria, malaria, malaria, and then maybe something else." She noted that there needs to be some system that suggests what the "something else" might be, either as part of the doctor's differential diagnosis or perhaps something in the laboratory that suggests what else should be tested. "But I agree the primary health care system is how we are likely going to pick up the potential beginning of a new pandemic," she said.

Elaborating on that, Hotez spoke of a metagenomics analysis of the viromes of individual mosquitoes caught in various places to create a surveillance ecology of arbovirus infections (Pan et al., 2024). Such an approach could make it possible, he suggested, to know what viruses mosquitoes are carrying in any given location throughout the world. "This would be useful not only for human health but also for animal health . . . and I don't think it's even going to be that expensive." "I would love to see an entire mapping exercise where we know where all the arboviruses are emerging, and I think this metagenomics approach is a very powerful way of doing it."

REFERENCES

Hayman, B., and S. Pagliusi. 2020. Emerging vaccine manufacturers are innovating for the next decade. *Vaccine X* 5:100066.
Hotez, P. J. 2021. *Preventing the Next Pandemic: Vaccine Diplomacy in a Time of Anti-Science*. Baltimore, MD: Johns Hopkins University Press.
Hotez, P. 2023. *Deadly Rise of Anti-Science: A Scientist's Warning*. Baltimore, MD: Johns Hopkins University Press.
Hotez, P. J., and A. D. LaBeaud. 2023. Yellow Jack's potential return to the American South. *New England Journal of Medicine* 389(16):1445–1447.
Hotez, P. J., K. O. Murray, and P. Buekens. 2014. The Gulf Coast: A new American underbelly of tropical diseases and poverty. *PLOS Neglected Tropical Diseases* 8(5):e2760.
Mehta, P., and P. J. Hotez. 2016. NTD and NCD co-morbidities: The example of dengue fever. *PLOS Neglected Tropical Diseases* 10(8):e0004619.
Murray, K. O., L. F. Rodriguez, E. Herrington, V. Kharat, N. Vasilakis, C. Walker, C. Turner, S. Khuwaja, R. Arafat, S. C. Weaver, D. Martinez, C. Kilborn, R. Bueno, and M. Reyna. 2013. Identification of dengue fever cases in Houston, Texas, with evidence of autochthonous transmission between 2003 and 2005. *Vector Borne Zoonotic Diseases* 13(12):835-845. https://doi.org/10.1089/vbz.2013.1413.

Pan, Y.-F., H. Zhao, Q.-Y. Gou, P.-B. Shi, J.-H. Tian, Y. Feng, K. Li, W.-H. Yang, D. Wu, G. Tang, B. Zhang, Z. Ren, S. Peng, G.-Y. Luo, S.-J. Le, G.-Y. Xin, J. Wang, X. Hou, M.-W. Peng, J.-B. Kong, X.-X. Chen, C.-H. Yang, S.-Q. Mei, Y.-Q. Liao, J.-X. Cheng, J. Wang, Chaolemen, Y.-H. Wu, J.-B. Wang, T. An, X. Huang, J.-S. Eden, J. Li, D. Guo, G. Liang, X. Jin, E.C. Holmes, B. Li, D. Wang, J. Li, W.-C. Wu, and M. Shi. 2024. Metagenomic analysis of individual mosquito viromes reveals the geographical patterns and drivers of viral diversity. *Nature Ecology & Evolution* 8(5):947-959. https://doi.org/10.1038/s41559-024-02365-0.

6

Arbovirus Spillover and Spread

Highlights

- The spillover and emergence of zoonotic pathogens can be analyzed in terms of four factors: spillover transmission from animals to humans, human-to-human transmissibility, the susceptibility of the human population, and the onward spread and connectivity. (Lloyd-Smith)
- Models using various types of data, including epidemiological data, environmental data, genomic data, clinical data, and experimental data, can be used to understand and predict the spread of emerging viruses. (Lloyd-Smith)
- CREATE-NEO (Coordinating Research on Emerging Arbovirus Threats Encompassing the Neotropics) is a network collecting data from surveillance sites and providing cutting-edge modeling approaches to dealing with emerging arboviruses. It also offers an example of how large amounts of data from disparate sources can be collected, organized, harmonized, analyzed, and made available to stakeholders. (Vasilakis)
- Risk assessment tools can be used to compare the risk of various arboviruses and identify which pose the greatest danger to public health and thus deserve the greatest scrutiny. (Pillai)

continued

- Implementation science provides the tools for more effectively putting into practice the novel strategies for the prevention and control of arboviral diseases that have been developed by public health and medical researchers. (Paz-Soldán)
- Behavioral and social scientists must be involved in efforts to modify behavior at the individual, community, and system levels as part of arboviral disease prevention and control. (Paz-Soldán)

NOTE: These points were made by the individual workshop speakers/participants identified above. They are not intended to reflect a consensus among workshop participants.

Peter Daszak of the EcoHealth Alliance, who moderated the first session on the workshop's second day, began by explaining that the sessions would examine innovative, forward-thinking approaches for future arbovirus mitigation. The first of the day's three sessions would look at arbovirus spillover and spread. Daszak stated that understanding arboviral emergence requires analyzing the pathogen's dynamics in its wildlife or livestock reservoir, understanding its movement through the human community, considering the environmental causes or drivers of those spillover events, and, finally, understanding the connections among human, animal, and environmental health, specifically with respect to arbovirus spillover and spread.

To bring those various perspectives to bear, four presenters would speak. First, Jamie Lloyd-Smith, professor in the Departments of Ecology and Evolutionary Biology and Computational Medicine at the University of California, Los Angeles, described using mathematical models to analyze zoonotic virus spillover and spread. Next, Nikos Vasilakis, vice chair for research in the Department of Pathology at the University of Texas Medical Branch, discussed CREATE-NEO (Coordinating Research on Emerging Arbovirus Threats Encompassing the Neotropics), a network collecting data and providing analytical tools to improve arbovirus prevention and control efforts. The third speaker, Segaran Pillai, director of the Office of Laboratory Safety at the U.S. Food and Drug Administration (FDA), spoke about using risk assessment tools to identify those arboviruses that pose the greatest risks to human populations. Finally, Valerie Paz-Soldán, associate professor in the Department of Tropical Medicine and Infectious Disease at Tulane University and director of Tulane's Health Office for Latin America in Lima, Peru, described how implementation science and behavioral and systems sciences can be used to maximize the effectiveness of new interventions against arbovirus spillover and spread.

ZOONOTIC DISEASE SPILLOVER AND EMERGENCE

Lloyd-Smith began by defining the reproductive number R, which is the average number of secondary cases infected by a typical case. Thus, R being greater than 1 is the threshold for sustained transmission of a pathogen.

Lloyd-Smith said, there are four key factors in considering emergence risk. The first is spillover from animals to humans, which "throws sparks of infection into the human population," he said. The second and third factors are human-to-human transmissibility and the susceptibility of the human population to the pathogen, which combine to determine the capacity for sustained spread. The transition to a larger epidemic or pandemic depends on the fourth factor: onward spread and connectivity in the human population plus the failure of any control measures.

The first factor, animal-to-human spillover transmission, is the defining characteristic of zoonoses, Lloyd-Smith said. Lloyd-Smith and colleagues proposed a general model for such spillover transmission that links the distribution and prevalence of infection in the reservoir hosts to the shedding of the pathogen into the environment, the possible pathogen survival or movement through the environment, and then the human behaviors that give rise to exposure to the pathogen as well as the host physical immune barriers that help determine the probability of an infection occurring.

Lloyd-Smith noted that these factors are dynamic, but when they align a spillover event can occur. The outcome of a spillover event can seem random, but studying the factors together can allow greater understanding of risk and possibly allow prediction of these events. Raina Plowright, one of Lloyd-Smith's colleagues who developed that framework, used it to unpack the factors governing the spillover of Hendra virus from bats in Australia (Plowright et al., 2015). That line of work culminated in a 2023 paper published in *Nature* that described a model that could predict the likelihood of spillover clusters from environmental data (Eby et al., 2023). Over the course of a decade, the model made two clear predictions of years that would have spillover clusters, Lloyd-Smith said, and those were indeed the 2 years in which spillover clusters occurred.

For the second factor, human-to-human transmissibility, the goal is to estimate transmissibility for pathogens that are threatening to emerge but have not yet led to an epidemic or pandemic, so data that could be used to analyze the validity of models are scarce. A key challenge occurs with subcritical pathogens, which transmit only weakly among humans so they lead only to small, self-limiting transmission chains. This means, Lloyd-Smith explained, that observed human cases are a mix of primary cases caused by infection from animals and secondary cases caused by human-to-human transmission. "The problem is," he said, "we don't generally know which are which." In response, Lloyd-Smith's team has developed model-based methods to estimate human-to-human R from real-world data (Blumberg and Lloyd-Smith, 2013a, b; Blumberg et al., 2014).

A parallel challenge that is important to assessing the risk of newly discovered viruses is using lab experiments, particularly from animal transmission studies, to infer something about human-to-human transmission. His team did a meta-analysis of ferret studies of flu transmission. (Buhnerkempe et al., 2015). They found that, statistically, if more than two-thirds of ferrets are infected via airborne spread, that strain is likely to be supercritical in humans—i.e., how well a flu strain spreads among laboratory ferrets via airborne transmission is an indicator of how strongly that strain is likely to spread through a human population.

The next frontier for this work, Lloyd-Smith said, is to get a clear understanding of the individual processes that go into a transmission event, including such things as virus shedding by the donor host, stability of the virus in the environment, dose–response dynamics, and immunity in the recipient, and use them to build a mechanistic model that can estimate transmission risk using virological data. "Then this can be tested against well-developed animal models for transmission and ultimately applied back in the human context," he said. The potential of this approach is hinted at by a model-based analysis that he and a team at the National Institutes of Health (NIH) performed early in the COVID-19 pandemic; they combined experimental data on the surface and aerosol stability of SARS-CoV-1 versus SARS-CoV-2 and drew on the known epidemiology of SARS-CoV-1 to predict the potential for airborne transmission and superspreading of the new virus. This was in March 2020, long before either airborne transmission or superspreading was recognized as a driver of the pandemic (van Doremalen et al., 2020).

The third factor, susceptibility of a population, is also a key issue. Novel viruses or zoonotic viruses that have never circulated widely among humans can face substantial preexisting population immunity. For instance, when children get their first exposure to seasonal flu, they get immunologically imprinted to that hemagglutinin group, giving them lifelong protection against avian flu viruses that have hemagglutinin from the same branch of the hemagglutinin family tree (Gostic et al., 2016). Because of this pattern, he said, population susceptibility can be computed and even projected over time from available data on demography and on seasonal flu incidence. A similar situation occurred with mpox, but in this case it was driven by vaccination against smallpox rather than by childhood exposure to a related virus. With the global eradication of smallpox in 1980, countries stopped smallpox vaccination programs, so cohorts of children started growing up who were not vaccinated against that virus and thus did not have resistance to mpox. Data on human mpox incidence in the Democratic Republic of Congo show this pattern clearly, with cases concentrated in those age groups born after the cessation of smallpox vaccination (Taube et al., 2023).

Turning to the fourth factor, onward spread and connectivity, Lloyd-Smith emphasized that after the initial spillover, a virus needs to establish a transmission chain. In earlier work, Lloyd-Smith and colleagues showed that substantial individual variation in transmissibility is ubiquitous across infectious diseases and that it plays a role in how a disease spreads (Lloyd-Smith et al., 2005). When transmissibility is highly variable, superspreading events can occur in which one individual is likely to infect many more individuals than an average infected person would. When individual variation in transmissibility is high, the spreading pathogen can give rise to explosive major outbreaks, but an introduction of the pathogen is also more likely to die out. As an example, he pointed to the original SARS virus, which was predicted to die out 75 percent of the time following an introduction, even though its R_0 of 3 is high enough to put it well into the dangerous domain (Lloyd-Smith et al., 2005).

The next hurdle to a viral introduction leading to an outbreak comes from the host population structure, he said. To cause a large epidemic, an outbreak must jump from its initial location to other regions. A key factor here, said Lloyd-Smith, is how often infected people move around relative to the infectious period. If movements are relatively rare, he said, "it doesn't matter how transmissible the pathogen is, it's going to burn out. It won't be able to penetrate the full population." Similarly, although traveler screening programs can affect the spread of a disease, the effectiveness of these programs will depend on the natural history of the infection, such as the incubation period, and on knowledge of risk factors, such as fever (Gostic et al., 2016). Unfortunately, Lloyd-Smith said, COVID-19 has a set of factors that mean that traveler screening programs will fail most of the time if it is the sole strategy in use.

In closing, Lloyd-Smith offered summarizing points. First, if emergence risk is broken into a series of constituent steps, each of those can be studied in turn. Then, he continued, "if we can think about the mechanisms that give rise to success of a pathogen in any one of these steps, that both enables us to study it more fruitfully and to come up with means of combating it." Upfront investments in modeling platforms and in data pipelines can help build capabilities for rapid response when new events occur and will also enable rational risk assessment that can guide longer term investment.

IMPLEMENTATION SCIENCE: OPERATIONALIZING ONE HEALTH DATA

Vasilakis is a principal investigator of CREATE-NEO,[1] which provides a network of surveillance sites in Central and South America along with cutting-edge modeling approaches with the goal of anticipating and

---

[1] See https://creid-network.org.

countering emerging arbovirus and SARS-CoV-2 threats. He spoke specifically about some of the tools used in CREATE-NEO to operationalize the growing masses of data as well as how those tools can be disseminated to various stakeholders and be used to ensure secure accessibility for all interested parties.

CREATE-NEO has several study sites across the Americas, and it applies a One Health approach in trying to understand the drivers behind viral emergence and outbreaks. It is a member of a global network of networks that generate "vast mountains of data that are coming from the different collection points," Vasilakis said. This amount of data raises many questions in terms of how it can best be handled, how to ensure ownership, how to ensure access, and how to make sure that credit goes to the people who have generated the data. Some have suggested, for example, that data should be stored in the originating institutions rather than in a centralized repository (CCGTT et al., 2017). This would ensure ownership, but there would need to be some way that the data could be accessed and analyzed by members of the global research community using widely available but secure methods under conditions that would ensure respect for the sensitivities of the originators of specific data.

Over the past 10 or 15 years, Vasilakis said, the number of public databases has greatly proliferated, and with the appearance of so many databases have come several challenges for those who would use them to address problems. First, the databases vary greatly in the type and scale of data and in the structure and size of the database. They vary in the quality of the data being collected, how often they are collected, and the level (local, country, global) at which they are collected. The databases also vary in the types of data collected. Regulatory and compliance issues may limit access to the data, and access may also be limited by more practical issues, such as how the data are stored (manual versus digital) and what language the database uses. Stakeholders in low- and middle-income countries may not be able to afford the necessary tools to access remote networks, for instance. These challenges together may hinder outbreak responses, Vasilakis said, because they may limit access to knowledge that could be crucial in recognizing a particular pathogen or learning lessons from previous experiences with it.

Next, Vasilakis provided a brief overview of some of the technologies CREATE-NEO uses to deal with the vast amounts of available data and meet the above challenges. There is great promise, he said, in semantic technology, which "collects data from different sources and assigns them machine-readable meanings." A critical component of semantic technology is knowledge graphs, which are used to connect disparate data with certain underlying elements across domains and skills. In creating a knowledge graph, primary data sources are identified first, then nodes are identified, and relationships between nodes are harmonized. This allows the knowledge graph to provide different outputs to the various stakeholders who would like to access those data and base decisions on them.

Vasilakis described work done by Barbara Han and Hailey Robertson to develop methods to use knowledge graphs for ecological systems, a major component of the CREATE-NEO research. Their work is intended to synthesize fragmented human, epidemiological, environmental, and zoonotic risk data; identify knowledge gaps; and generate hypotheses about, for example, what spillover events occur and what their frequency is. Such work depends critically on open data sources, he continued, but with open access comes several other issues that must be addressed, such as the issue of ownership and how contributors of data can be recognized and rewarded.

Vasilakis then described work by Peter McCaffrey, a physician at the University of Texas Medical Branch, to develop a "data lakehouse" that is used for primary storage, access, and interrogation of data. Individual collaborators deposit data of various types—metadata, clinical data, geolocation files, and so on—directly into an Amazon Web Services S3 storage system. In essence, Vasilakis said, the system integrates and assesses the data that are input and provides meaningful outputs for the various stakeholders. The data can be of a wide variety of types—radiology images, clinical notes and interpretations from clinicians, lab results, and more. The various stakeholders of CREATE-NEO, including international policy makers, private researchers, clinicians, and people who help facilitate the operations, can access all those data, analyze the data, repurpose them for other analyses and, in general, obtain useful information out of them.

Looking to the future, Vasilakis said that there are many gaps remaining. Stakeholders must be able to claim ownership while facilitating data accessibility, he said. Removing barriers to data sharing will also be important. One of the ways that the CREATE-NEO network has approached that accessibility challenge is with collaboration agreements and memoranda of understanding that provide a foundation for sharing data. Communication with the stakeholders is also vital, he added, since they must understand and appreciate the responsibility and accountability that come with sharing the data, such as giving credit to and being respectful of the ownership of the individual contributors.

Finally, Vasilakis said, there needs to be comprehensive and effective programs for the acquisition of data as well as for stakeholder engagement. It will be important to ensure that the benefits of using the data from this network, whether the discovery of a new vaccine or better tools for clinical care, are distributed equitably and benefit the original contributors of the data.

RANKING DISEASE THREATS

Pillai described in detail a method he developed to rank the seriousness of threats from different arboviruses and what the rankings reveal when viewed in different ways. He offered the caveat that "this is still a work in progress and will require some further refinement upon consultation with my colleagues, who are experts in this area."

He began with some context. Globally, more than 25 percent of human infectious diseases are vector-borne diseases, and these diseases contribute to more than 2.5 million deaths each year. Mosquitoes and ticks are the main vectors, along with sandflies and midges. To date, more than 550 arboviruses have been described, of which about 50 cause disease in animals and more than 130 cause infections and diseases in humans and animals. It is important to periodically conduct risk assessments to inform activities designed to prevent, prepare for, and respond to arbovirus outbreaks.

To rank the disease threats posed by various arboviruses, Pillai used a standard multistep approach. It begins by clearly defining the key factors that will be used in the analysis and establishing the criteria for scoring. The next step is data collection, where all the available scientific data and information that can be used to score the criteria are gathered. With that information, a score is assigned to each virus on each criterion using the established scoring scheme. Next, weights are assigned based on importance of the criteria. Then the analysis is performed using a one-dimensional or two-dimensional approach with and without the assigned weights so that the different outcomes can be compared.

Additionally, Pillai performs a decision support framework analysis, which is "a very simple logic-tree approach, asking a series of critical questions that will either move the virus to the next stage or drop it out from any further analysis." Pillai's risk assessment included a total of 54 viruses that cause disease in humans: 14 *Flaviviridae*, 13 *Togaviridae*, 2 *Reoviridae*, 4 *Rhabdoviridae*, and 21 *Bunyaviridae*. Three key factors were considered in determining the risk score of each virus: transmission, consequence, and mitigation (Figure 6-1). The transmission factor considered the vectors involved, the reservoir of hosts other than humans, and the disease/vector distribution pattern. The consequence factor included vulnerable populations, status of immunity, total number of cases per year, severity of symptoms, the case fatality rate, and long-term health impacts. The mitigation factor examined the availability of rapid diagnostics, availability of medical countermeasures, burden on public health care and vector control measures

In scoring the viruses, Pillai explained, each criterion was scored on a scale of 0 to 10 for each virus. For example, in the case of fatality rate, a rate greater than 25 percent would get a score of 10, 20–24 would get a score of 8, and anything close to 0 percent would get a score of 0. Each

Methodology Uses a Multi-Criteria Decision Analysis Approach to Derive the Agent Risk

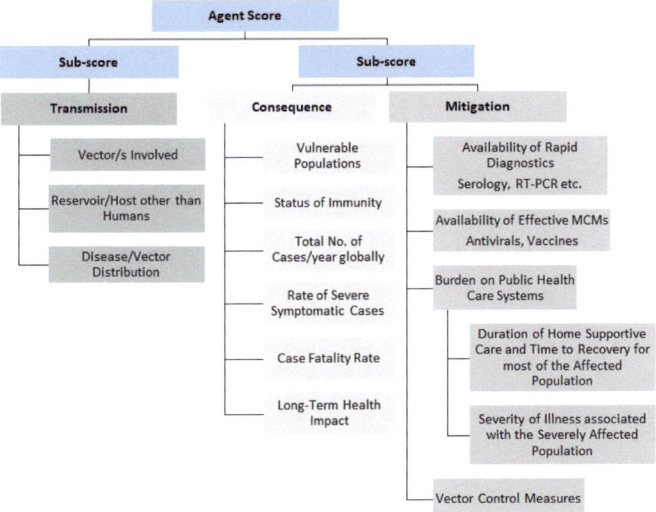

FIGURE 6-1 The factors in determining the risk score for each virus.
SOURCE: Presented by Segaran Pillai on December 13, 2023.

criterion was assigned a weight, and the overall score for a virus was determined by summing the individual weighted criterion scores for that virus.

Displaying the scores in a two-dimensional plot as opposed to a one-dimensional plot allows additional insight on risk ranking and clarifies distinctions among viruses that rank in the middle, Pillai said. This plot elucidates where the virus scored in terms of transmission versus its score in terms of consequences plus mitigation. Weighing the criteria provided better separation of the agents in both the one-dimensional and the two-dimensional plots. In the two-dimensional plots, the upper right quadrant contains viruses with both a high transmission score and a high impact score, the lower right quadrant has viruses with a low transmission score but high consequences, and so on (Figure 6-2). Again, one can determine thresholds of interest, although in the two-dimensional case, the thresholds will be in the shape of an L and everything above and to the right of the L are beyond the threshold.

Next, Pillai shared the results of evaluating the same set of arboviruses with the decision support framework instead of the risk scores. The various factors considered in that framework were agent qualification, transmission, disease, vulnerable populations, pathogenicity and severity

Scoring Results

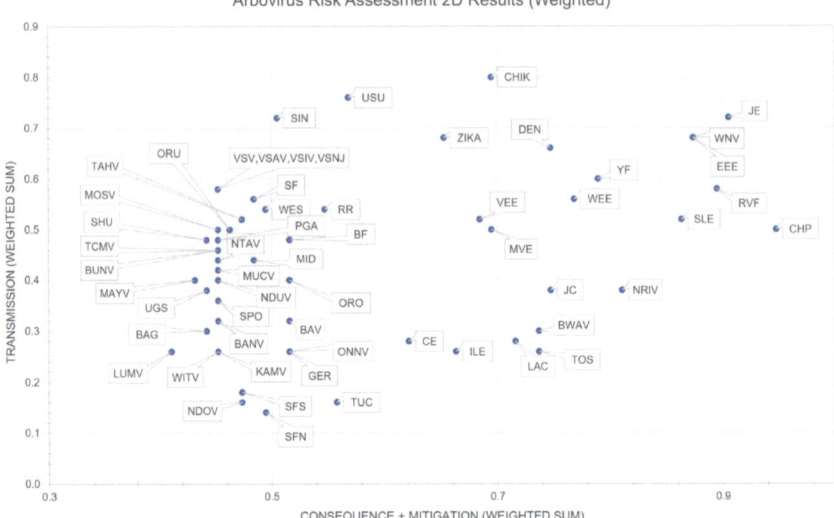

FIGURE 6-2 Weighted scores in the arbovirus risk assessment displayed in two dimensions.
NOTES: Arboviruses in top right box indicate viruses with both a high consequence score and a high impact score. CHPV = Chandipura virus; EEEV = Eastern equine encephalitis virus; JEV = Japanese encephalitis virus; RVFV = Rift Valley fever virus; SLEV = St. Louis encephalitis virus; WEEV = Western equine encephalitis; WNV = West Nile virus; YFV = yellow fever virus.
SOURCE: Presented by Segaran Pillai on December 13, 2023.

of illness, hospitalization rates, the availability of rapid diagnostics and medical countermeasures, the morbidity and mortality rates associated with the pathogen or the disease, and, finally, the public health impact. In comparing the results from the scoring analysis and the decision support framework analysis, Pillai said, he found that the two-dimensional weighted scores and the decision support framework identified nearly the same tier 1 and tier 2 risk groups. Among the four different ways of analyzing the risk assessment scores—weighted versus unweighted and one-dimensional versus two-dimensional—differences appeared in, for example, exactly which viruses made it into tier 1, but in general the results were mostly consistent. "Overall," he said, "what we are observing is Japanese encephalitis virus, Eastern equine encephalitis virus, Chandipura virus, West Nile virus, Rift Valley Fever Virus, Saint Louis encephalitis virus, yellow fever virus, and

Western equine encephalitis virus seem to consistently fall in the tier 1 risk group of arboviruses."

In conclusion, Pillai said that the analysis should be seen mainly as a tool rather than as a single result. "If any of the data change, those data can then be applied to the scoring scheme and applied back into the risk assessment tool and replot the entire graph," he said. "So, it's not a static assessment, but it's a very fluid, very dynamic process of doing risk assessment." It allows one to respond very quickly to changes in circumstances with a new analysis and new understanding in terms of which viruses pose the greatest risk to public health.

BEHAVIOR MANAGEMENT TO PREVENT SPILLOVER AND SPREAD

Modifying human behavior can play an important role in preventing and controlling outbreaks of arboviral disease, Paz-Soldán said. Behavior change matters, she explained, because it enables the implementation of novel and evidence-based strategies in diverse epidemiological, geographic, and cultural contexts. It is important to consider behavior change at the individual level and at the community systems level when implementing arbovirus prevention and control efforts, Paz-Soldán continued. In studying what works to create such behavioral change, she said, randomized controlled trials are not necessarily the optimal choice because an innovation may not be put into practice the same way it was done in a trial. So, she concluded, research should focus on how programs are implemented in real settings with real challenges and real bottlenecks and on how to deal with these challenges as they emerge.

Paz-Soldán highlighted that it is important to consider how to implement approaches such as new vaccines and new vector-control strategies that are showing effectiveness. This is where implementation science fits in, she said. "Implementation science . . . is the science that translates evidence into policy and into practice. And it takes into consideration the fact that context matters, that the different levels in stakeholders matter, and that the processes by which we apply these innovations matter."

To illustrate the important factors in implementation research and how they fit together, Paz-Soldán referred to the Consolidated Framework for Implementation Research (Damschroder et al., 2022) (Figure 6-3). The framework begins with "the what," or the innovation that needs to be implemented. Much of the funding in this area focuses on developing effective strategies for arboviral disease prevention and control, she said, but it is also important to think about how these strategies are put into practice. Finally, one must consider the individuals involved in the implementation

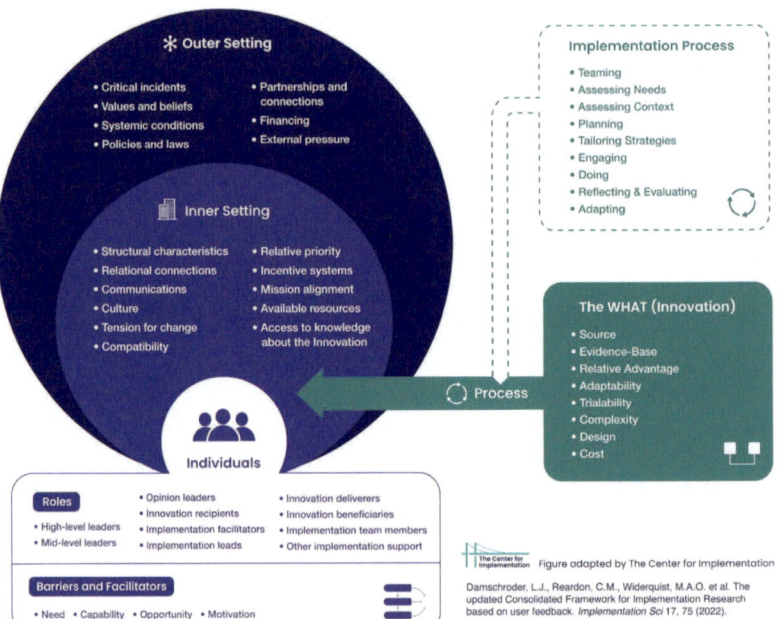

FIGURE 6-3 Consolidated framework for implementation research.
SOURCES: Presented by Valerie A. Paz-Soldán on December 13, 2023. From the Consolidated Framework for Implementation Research (CFIR) 2.0, 2022. Adapted from *The updated Consolidated Framework for Implementation Research based on user feedback*, by Damschroder, L.J., Reardon, C.M., Widerquist, M.A.O. et al., 2022, *Implementation Sci* 17, 75. Copyright by The Center for Implementation. https://thecenterforimplementation.com/toolbox/cfir; CC BY 4.0.

and the environments in which they operate, from the individuals who deliver the innovation, those who receive it, and to various leaders and facilitators and beneficiaries.

Implementation scientists need to observe and consider all of the different aspects of implementation in the figure, Paz-Soldán said. In the case of "the what," for instance, one must consider the evidence base behind the innovation as well as its complexity, design, cost, and relative advantage over other strategies. These factors help determine which innovations to prioritize and which should get funded in a specific country or setting.

The environments involved with the innovation begins with those individuals living in an area affected by the arbovirus and targeted by an intervention. The individual's beliefs about the intervention or how they perceive it to work or not work is important to consider. Next there are people in what Paz-Soldán called the "inner setting," which includes those involved in primary health care and those local or regional health authorities who need to decide how to operationalize the intervention. Finally, there is the "outer setting," which includes such things as the policies and regulations coming from the national level, international guidance, partnerships, and funding.

As an example of the sort of outer setting that must be considered, Paz-Soldán spoke about the situation in her country of Peru, which has had seven presidents and 16 ministers of health in the past 8 years. "The ministers of health have had an average, I think, of 143 days in office," she said, "so, they are not thinking long term." They are thinking about what they can be doing in 2 or 3 months that can make a difference. Furthermore, if something goes wrong, the minister at the time will likely be the scapegoat. Thus, it is a major challenge to convince the health minister to use their limited time in office to put into place the evidence-based strategies that have been identified by scientists as working in much less challenging settings.

The inner setting offers equally vexing challenges. Even if the minister of health instructs local directors to adopt a certain policy, the local officials are faced with all sorts of difficulties, such as unclear strategy, time, funding, and uncertainty of responsibilities, Paz-Soldán said. Conflicts of interest must also be considered. "You want to call it corruption, you want to call it conflict of interest," she said, "but a lot of times the insecticide that we decide upon is because your friend who's working in this lab is selling that one. That's the reality of the situation."

Finally, at the individual level, implementation scientists must think about what is realistic to expect in terms of changing individual behavior. Is it reasonable to expect people to regularly wear masks for months at a time or to apply insecticide every day when it is costly and irritates the skin and eyes? People can come to view diseases as inevitable. And sometimes when the government takes steps, such as instituting a vector-control program, individuals may decide that it is not their responsibility and the government will take care of it.

To address these challenges, implementation science has strategies for adapting an innovation to a particular context, but this requires pre-implementation preparation, such as developing protocols, creating a timeline, and determining who will have responsibilities for various tasks. Such preparation needs to take place at both the national level and the regional level, Paz-Soldán added. Furthermore, the workers need to consider what data streams and information will be available and how to identify where bottlenecks are occurring, and they should continuously monitor and evaluate the situation. A key aspect of all of this is the question of whose responsibility it is to plan, adapt, and implement these new strategies and who should be contacted when the program hits a snag.

The positive message to take away from this, Paz-Soldán said, is that implementation science does offer an effective approach to dealing with these various challenges. However, it is handicapped by a lack of funding. Foundations, for instance, have focused mostly on developing evidence-based interventions. "You can spend millions of dollars on that one innovation," she said, "but it's rare to even give $20,000 to a social scientist trying to pilot how this innovation can be made sustainable practice in a community." The NIH now has a funding mechanism through which to fund implementation science, she said, and that gives her hope that there will be more focus on the process by which innovations are put into practice.

In conclusion, she said, behavioral and social scientists need to be part of encouraging the individual-, community-, and system-level behavioral change needed to enable arboviral disease prevention and control. It will be crucial to take a more transdisciplinary approach to integrate social and behavioral scientists into the overall arbovirus mitigation efforts. Funding should focus on behavior change as well as on the development of evidence-based vector control, vaccines, and treatments. And education in this area should emphasize developing researchers trained in a transdisciplinary approach who look at all the different parts of the system and focus on keeping all the cogs in that machine working together smoothly.

To close, she offered an African proverb: If you want to go fast, go alone; if you want to go far, go accompanied. "We must work together towards those challenges."

DISCUSSION

In the discussion session following the presentations, Lloyd-Smith was asked how his models deal with the fact that each spillover event involving an emerging disease seems to be unique and complex and whether findings from his models can be applied broadly across emerging diseases.

Lloyd-Smith responded that that complexity was one of the motivations for his team's effort to determine the minimal set of factors needed to line up for a spillover event to occur. His goal is to work with the rich descriptions of various spillover events and extract the details that answer the specific questions asked by the model. "The hope is that we can at least find the commonalities among all these different rich anecdotes and particular events," he said. He noted that some spillover events—such as the West African Ebola outbreak or the origins of COVID-19—are of very high consequence, while many other spillover events occur regularly by the same mechanisms but without serious consequences. "One of the important questions, I think, is the degree to which we can learn about the processes which may give rise to those rare high-impact events by studying the more common ones," he said. "Can we learn about the science of spillover from things that are spilling over all the time?" The goal, he concluded, is to apply this systematic approach to synthesize evidence and then identify the common themes and turn that into actionable interventions.

Next, Marcos Espinal asked Paz-Soldán about the issue of building trust and engagement with communities, particularly those in low- and middle-income countries. Trust is not built overnight, Paz-Soldán replied. "I think it has really helped that I am Peruvian. I live in Peru. I was born and raised there, and I spent the last 20 years living near the communities." However, she continued, it is also vital to identify local champions, nurture those relationships, and then rely on those champions to influence their communities and help move things forward. It is also important to give back to communities when possible. Finally, she added that the trust low- and middle-income countries had in the Global North was damaged during the COVID-19 pandemic because of the lack of equity in vaccine distribution.

Next, a workshop participant asked Vasilakis about the best way to ensure long-term funding for databases. Vasilakis acknowledged that funders often lose interest in funding databases once they have been established, but he said that the CREATE-NEO network "offers a pathway for maintaining those databases in either centralized or individualized databases that may be able to be assessed, given the widespread interactions and/or collaborations across various entities." CREATE has established relationships among many different networks, he said, and it should be possible to maintain those relationships over long periods of time with the contributions of individual stakeholders. As for the databases themselves, maintaining them and having access to them is crucial, he said, and the various stakeholders recognize that. Ultimately, "it takes advocacy on our part to make the appropriate [funders] fully appreciate the long-term utility and maintenance of those databases."

Another workshop participant asked Paz-Soldán about continuity in health authorities in low- and middle-income countries, getting funding for the "last mile" of implementing arbovirus control programs, and how to argue for behavioral change, given that the available evidence indicates that behavioral factors generally account for no more than 20 percent of the explanation for the success of programs.

Concerning the first question about fast turnover and information that is lost, Paz-Soldán acknowledged that being something she struggles with. One approach she has considered is creating partnerships between academia and mid-level technicians at the health institutions who are less likely to turn over quickly to make it more likely that any lessons learned become part of the institutional memory. Ultimately, she said, researchers should be studying that issue of sustainability and coming up with strategies for building it up. On the issue of the last mile, she said that the implementation science grants that have been gaining traction have created an environment in which there is a greater appreciation of the importance of the last steps in putting an innovation in place. This, in turn, may make it easier to get funding for the last mile and make sure that the new innovation becomes a sustainable practice in the community.

Finally, she acknowledged that there have been many theories of behavior change and many of them have not worked. "Human behavior is very complex," she said. "There are so many different levels that maybe 20 percent is actually not that bad." The key is that when one is thinking about arboviral disease prevention and control, the entire system needs to be considered. There will always be value in considering the specifics of human behavior and culture in each place, but it should only be a part of a larger, more comprehensive approach that addresses the systems.

Lloyd-Smith was then asked how the data analyses used to predict the risk of viral outbreaks could be used to encourage people to take preventive measures against something they cannot see, particularly since if the predictions are accurate and the preventive measures are effective, outbreaks would not occur. One approach, he said, would be to carefully document pathogens that are constantly spilling over and produce a reliable estimate of their risk, "so that when you do put in interventions and hopefully reduce that risk, you're able to make a reliable quantitative assessment of the impact of those interventions." Something similar could be done with viruses that have less spillover but pose the risk of a major epidemic when they do get into the human population, Lloyd-Smith said. Daszak added that if economists could provide a dollar value for the human illnesses and deaths prevented by the control efforts, that might make for an even more compelling argument.

REFERENCES

Blumberg, S., and J. O. Lloyd-Smith. 2013a. Inference of R_0 and transmission heterogeneity from the size distribution of stuttering chains. *PLOS Computational Biology* 9(5):e1002993.

Blumberg, S., and J. O. Lloyd-Smith. 2013b. Comparing methods for estimating R_0 from the size distribution of subcritical transmission chains. *Epidemics* 5(3):131–145.

Blumberg, S., W. T. Enanoria, J. O. Lloyd-Smith, T. M. Lietman, and T. C. Porco. 2014. Identifying postelimination trends for the introduction and transmissibility of measles in the United States. *American Journal of Epidemiology* 179(11):1375–1382.

Buhnerkempe, M. G., K. Gostic, M. Park, P. Ahsan, J. A. Belser, and J. O. Lloyd-Smith. 2015. Mapping influenza transmission in the ferret model to transmission in humans. *eLife* 4:e07969.

CCGTT (Clinical Cancer Genome Task Team of the Global Alliance for Genomics and Health), M. Lawler, D. Haussler, L. L. Siu, M. A. Haendel, J. A. McMurry, B. M. Knoppers, S. J. Chanock, F. Calvo, B. T. The, G. Walia, I. Banks, P. P. Yu, L. M. Staudt, and C. L. Sawyers. 2017. Sharing clinical and genomic data on cancer—The need for global solutions. *New England Journal of Medicine* 376(21):2006–2009.

CFIR (The Consolidated Framework for Implementation Research 2.0). 2022. Adapted from "The updated Consolidated Framework for Implementation Research based on user feedback," by L. J. Damschroder, C. M. Reardon, M. A. O. Widerquist, et al., 2022. *Implementation Science* 17:75. Copyright by The Center for Implementation. https://thecenterforimplementation.com/toolbox/cfir (accessed June 5, 2024).

Damschroder, L. J., C. M. Reardon, M. A. O. Widerquist, and J. Lowery. 2022. The updated Consolidated Framework for Implementation Research based on user feedback. *Implementation Science* 17(1):75. https://doi.org/10.1186/s13012-022-01245-0.

Eby, P., A. J. Peel, A. Hoegh, W. Madden, J. R. Giles, P. J. Hudson, and R. K. Plowright. 2023. Pathogen spillover driven by rapid changes in bat ecology. *Nature* 613(7943):340–344.

Gostic, K. M., M. Ambrose, M. Worobey, and J. O. Lloyd-Smith. 2016. Potent protection against H5N1 and H7N9 influenza via childhood hemagglutinin imprinting. *Science* 354(6313):722–726.

Lloyd-Smith, J. O., S. J. Schreiber, P. E. Kopp, and W. M. Getz. 2005. Superspreading and the effect of individual variation on disease emergence. *Nature* 438(7066):355–359.

Plowright, R. K., P. Eby, P. J. Hudson, I. L. Smith, D. Westcott, W. L. Bryden, D. Middleton, P. A. Reid, R. A. McFarlane, G. Martin, G. M. Tabor, L. F. Skerratt, D. L. Anderson, G. Crameri, D. Quammen, D. Jordan, P. Freeman, L. F. Wang, J. H. Epstein, G. A. Marsh, N. Y. Kung, and H. McCallum. 2015. Ecological dynamics of emerging bat virus spillover. *Proceedings of the Royal Society B: Biological Sciences* 282(1798):20142124.

Plowright, R. K., C. R. Parrish, H. McCallum, P. J. Hudson, A. I. Ko, A. L. Graham, and J. O. Lloyd-Smith. 2017. Pathways to zoonotic spillover. *Nature Reviews Microbiology* 15(8):502–510.

Taube, J. C., E. C. Rest, J. O. Lloyd-Smith, and S. Bansal. 2023. The global landscape of smallpox vaccination history and implications for current and future orthopoxvirus susceptibility: A modelling study. *The Lancet Infectious Diseases* 23(4):454–462. https://doi.org/10.1016/S1473-3099(22)00664-8.

van Doremalen, N., T. Bushmaker, D. H. Morris, M. G. Holbrook, A. Gamble, B. N. Williamson, A. Tamin, J. L. Harcourt, N. J. Thornburg, S. I. Gerber, J. O. Lloyd-Smith, E. de Wit, and V. J. Munster. 2020. Aerosol and surface stability of SARS-CoV-2 as compared with SARS-CoV-1. *New England Journal of Medicine* 382(16):1564–1567.

7

Urban Development and Management

Highlights

- *Aedes aegypti* mosquitoes are the major carrier of the most important arboviruses, such as dengue, Zika, yellow fever, and chikungunya, so it makes sense to focus prevention and control efforts on these mosquitoes, particularly in urban areas, where the risks of transmission are highes. (Lindsay)
- "Building-out" interventions, which focus on changing the built environment in ways that make it less hospitable to mosquito breeding and create barriers to human contact by mosquitoes, are an effective way of reducing the transmission of arboviruses in urban areas. (Lindsay)
- Urban areas will become an increasingly important area for vector-control efforts as they grow in the coming decades, particularly in those parts of the urban areas occupied by slums, which have poorer infrastructure and health care. (Alabaster)
- Vector-control efforts and public health programs need to be tailored to the urban area in question; a "one size fits all" approach does not work. (Alabaster)
- A two-pronged strategy where short-term pilot projects demonstrate the value of a particular approach and influence the design of larger, longer-term projects can be effective in convincing cities to incorporate new vector-control techniques. (Alabaster)

continued

- Experience in Singapore shows that reshaping the built environment—in this case, moving a significant percentage of the population from low-lying slums to high-rise apartments—can have a major effect on the transmission of arboviruses. (Ooi)
- In Africa, a new mosquito species that carries malaria, *Anopheles stephensi*, is spreading in urban areas. Because it often shares its larval habitats with *Aedes aegypti*, there are opportunities here for integrated surveillance and control of both types of mosquitoes with benefits for both malaria and arboviral diseases. (Wilson)

NOTE: These points were made by the individual workshop speakers/participants identified above. They are not intended to reflect a consensus among workshop participants.

Linda S. Lloyd of San Diego State University served as moderator of the workshop's sixth session, which discussed how best to control the spread of arboviral diseases in urban areas. The panel's first speaker was Steve Lindsay, a public health entomologist and epidemiologist at Durham University, who discussed ways to modify urban infrastructures to limit populations of *Aedes* mosquitoes and their ability to transmit viruses. Next, Graham Alabaster, the director of UN–Habitat at the Geneva office of the United Nations (UN), spoke about how to design and implement vector-control projects designed for specific urban areas. Dr. Eng Eong Ooi, a professor in the emerging infectious diseases at the Duke-National University of Singapore Medical School, offered a case study of how Singapore limited the transmission of arboviruses, such as dengue, through a combination of vector control programs and replacing most of its slum neighborhoods with high-rise buildings developed by the government. Finally, Anne Wilson, an infectious disease epidemiologist at the Liverpool School of Tropical Medicine, described the appearance of a new malaria vector in Africa, *Anopheles stephensi*, and suggested that there is an opportunity to combine surveillance and control efforts for malaria with those for arboviral diseases.

VISION FOR BUILDING *AEDES* OUT

Lindsay spoke about "building out Aedes," which is the approach of modifying urban environments to control the spread of arboviruses by limiting breeding opportunities for *Aedes aegypti* mosquitoes.

In recent decades, Lindsay said, there have been huge increases in the number of dengue cases around the world, mainly in the tropics and subtropics, and there have also been growing numbers of Zika, yellow fever, and chikungunya cases. All these diseases are transmitted by *Aedes aegypti*. This species is the world's most efficient vector of viruses, and it is distributed throughout most of the world's tropical and subtropical regions, including much of South America, Central America, and the Southeastern United States as well as subtropical Africa, India, and Southeast Asia. It was originally a forest mosquito, breeding in tree holes, but it was able to spread around the world because its eggs are highly resilient and it adapted to breeding in small containers of water. "It is an extraordinarily adaptable, invasive species," he said. In modern cities, *Aedes aegypti* will lay its eggs wherever there is standing water. Most commonly this means in open containers where people are storing water because the local water supply is not reliable, in discarded tires with collected rainwater, and bits of waste in which water sits.

Lindsay's approach to controlling arbovirus transmission is built on limiting the numbers of *Aedes aegypti* mosquitoes. He focuses on urban areas because this is where most of the arbovirus transmission problem exists today and because, if it is not addressed, the problem of arbovirus transmission in urban areas will get much worse in the future. "Urban population will double by 2050," he said, "and nearly seven out of ten people in this world will live in cities" (World Bank, 2023). Though this is a challenge, the urban population explosion also offers an opportunity, he continued, as 60 percent of the urban areas that will be there in 2050 have not yet been built. "[This is] important because it presents an opportunity to guide the design of towns and cities around the world because most of this increase is not going to be in the cities that are already built, but it's going to be in what we now think of as secondary towns."

Focusing efforts on cities rather than countries can also be effective because cities are recognized as engines of change, he said. Epidemiologists and researchers can work with mayors to show that by taking steps to reduce *Aedes aegypti* populations, they can provide a healthy environment for workers and improve the economy, Lindsay said.

Lindsay's group's approach to controlling mosquitoes is two-pronged. The first prong is enhanced integrated control, which he described as a fusion of classical entomological and clinical approaches, including traditional surveillance tools combined with the appropriate responses when signs of the vector or the disease are spotted. The second prong is what Lindsay referred to as "building out," or changing the environment to be less conducive to the spread of *Aedes aegypti*. "Essentially what we're trying to do is prevent small bodies of water [from] accumulating and doing something to reduce biting rates and biting indoors as well," he said. One way to do this, for instance, is to provide reliable pipe water. If people know that they can turn on the tap and water will come out, they will have no reason to store water. It will also be important to remove trash, improve drainage, close water containers, remove gutters, build concrete structures that are impervious to mosquitoes, and make sure that homes have screening. Lindsay noted the importance of building clean cities where there is less surface water. Most importantly, he continued, the interventions need to be tailored to local conditions. Building out *Aedes* should be a city-led approach with dynamic city leaders who can pull people together and break down silos.

Lindsay outlined an approach that relies on three foundations: community involvement and support, a health department that works across sectors, and research and development. Community involvement is important not only because the approach requires getting buy-in from the community but also because the community can make suggestions about what local innovations might be appropriate when coming up with solutions to problems. Having health departments working across sectors is about breaking down barriers, Lindsay said, with the ultimate goal of having collaborations between health departments and those in the built environment. Continued research and development are also necessary, noting that greater investment to assess efficacy of interventions is essential. This approach involves distinct types of actions: effective surveillance, monitoring, and evaluation of interventions; mosquito control by means of reducing breeding sites, engineering the built environment, and using pesticides; and the use of vaccines, antivirals, and case management to control viral transmission in the human population. The combination of these actions would, he said, lead to effective, locally adapted control of *Aedes*-transmitted viral disease.

The approach fits well with the UN sustainable development goals created in 2015, Lindsay said. Goal 3, for example, is good health and well-being. Goal 6 is clean water and sanitation. Goal 11 is sustainable cities and communities. "We need to think about the control of dengue and other viral diseases as a sustainable cities or towns [issue]," he said. Goal 13 is climate action, which is particularly relevant because climate change could increase the range of *Aedes aegypti* and may also prolong the mosquitoes' season, exacerbating future epidemics. A secondary effect of climate change may be increased droughts, which could lead to people being more likely to store water in open containers and providing more habitat for *Aedes aegypti*.

Lindsay acknowledged that the building-out approach would be expensive and outside the usual bounds of public health, but there are already examples of cities planning future growth with various forward-looking objectives in mind. He pointed, for instance, to the Making Cities Resilient 2030 initiative, which involves a collection of agencies who assist cities in making their communities more resilient and sustainable (UNDRR, n.d.). Given that such a network of cities focused on future sustainability issues already exists, it would make sense to reach out to the people in this network and explain that there is another major environmental problem—that of *Aedes*-transmitted viral diseases—that their cities need to be defended from. "These networks exist, but they don't understand the language and we're not tapping at their doors, and we should be," Lindsay said. "There is an opportunity here." Lindsay highlighted the importance of a city leader-led approach that engages communities and develops innovative mitigation strategies that meet health, sustainability, and economic needs of the city.

PUBLIC HEALTH IN URBAN ENVIRONMENTS

Alabaster spoke in general about the factors affecting public health in urban environments and what can be done to improve public health. Across the globe, more and more people are living in cities. By 2030, projections indicate that about 5 billion people will live in cities, up from just more than 2 billion in 1990. In the coming years it will not be just the bigger cities that are growing, but medium-size cities will also grow extremely fast.

Urban areas are susceptible to issues relating to health and environment for a variety of reasons, he said. Many of them lack the necessary capacities in the health sector, and the process of urbanization is extremely inefficient. This leads to large unplanned areas, which are referred to by various names in different parts of the world—slums, bustees, favelas, and so on—and in many countries, these areas are where much of the workforce live.

The result, Alabaster continued, is that even in the more developed regions of the world, many cities have an underclass of people who lack access to basic services. It is most pronounced in sub-Saharan Africa and Central Asia and Southern Asia, where approximately half of the urban population was living in slums in 2020. "Those are the people who don't have access to services," he said, such as health services, water, sanitation, and waste management.

Although worldwide the percentage of urban populations living in slums has decreased significantly over the past 20 years (from 64 percent to 50 percent in sub-Saharan Africa, for instance), slum populations are still increasing. Many people are driven by conflict or climate change to migrate to large cities, and they generally end up in the low-income areas. Alabaster said he and colleagues have studied the capacity of the slums in these cities, "and it's reaching saturation." Thus, they anticipate further reduced access to health services and increased incidences of disease in these areas.

The COVID-19 pandemic offered an indication of what could be expected in urban areas hit by an arbovirus outbreak, he said. The pandemic magnified existing inequities in health care in urban settings, with those who had poorer access to health care before the pandemic feeling the effects of those inequities to a much greater degree during the pandemic. A variety of factors governed the varying impacts of COVID-19,

Alabaster said. One such factor was overcrowding. "It's not just about density," he explained. "It's about overcrowding of services and access to services." Comorbidities also played a major role. In the Global North, the most important comorbidities during the pandemic were noncommunicable diseases, while in the south they were other communicable diseases, particularly vector-borne diseases. Differences in treatment-seeking behavior played a role in how COVID-19 affected people differently, as did demographics. Furthermore, cities were very different in their ability to respond; some of the cities that did well in the pandemic were the ones that had effective triaging systems and isolated the most vulnerable populations early on. City governments are responsible for implementing national policy, but they are also the ones who best know their community, Alabaster noted. Because of these differences among cities, a "one-size-fits-all" response to an epidemic or pandemic is not likely to be widely effective, Alabaster said. It is vital to understand the specifics of an individual community in order to deliver effective services, and that in turn requires accumulating a great deal of spatially disaggregated data—not just on the populations but also on their access to services. During the COVID-19 pandemic, the UN developed a dashboard for cities that focused on city statistics, rather than national statistics, which contained data provided by local health departments. This might be something that could be usefully applied to arboviral diseases, he suggested, because it could provide better spatial information on an outbreak.

Alabaster said that one can think about urban areas as providing opportunities rather than challenges. For example, 60 percent of the urban areas that will exist in 2050 have not yet been built, so making sure those areas are designed and built to promote better health and greater resistance to the spread of arboviral and other diseases could make a huge difference to the people who will be living in them. Furthermore, cities offer opportunities because they can be shaped by strong local civic leaders. Such leaders are the "missing middle"—they are well placed to work with the national government, and they are the ones with the best knowledge of their communities. And it is at the local level that many policies important to public health—such as policies for solid waste management—are determined. "Many of the things that we know we can do to control the disease vectors are the responsibility of municipal authorities," Alabaster said.

One key to convincing city leaders of the importance of arboviral disease mitigation, he said, is to emphasize that the methods used to deal with these diseases will be effective with other cities as well. In the Kenyan city of Kisumu during the COVID-19 pandemic, enteric diseases almost disappeared because of the hygiene methods imposed for COVID. That was a "marvelous learning experience" for the city officials in Kisumu because it helped them see how valuable such methods were to improved health outside of COVID. City leaders must see the health and economic benefits of making environmental modifications, such as piped water and waste disposal, he said.

An important tool for convincing city leaders and urban planners of the importance of these steps is the use of pilot demonstrations. Providing short-term "quick wins" in things like vector control can make it more likely that cities will adopt some of the effective approaches in their more long-term plans for urban expansion. In November 2021, the World Health Organization (WHO) and UN–Habitat launched the Healthy Cities, Healthy People initiative, which is designed to get mayors and other local authorities to understand and invest in a health-promoting infrastructure. One goal of the Healthy Cities, Healthy People initiative is to generate these small-scale pilot projects and encourage cities to take that approach in their longer-term infrastructure projects. It may be challenging to find funding to carry out short-term trials and demonstrations in some neighborhoods of the city, but once the value of the new approach has been established, Alabaster said, "it becomes a relatively easy step to upscale and to expand into other areas of the city." In conclusion, Alabaster summarized what is needed to move urban areas in a direction that is more resistant to arboviral diseases. The first step is to understand the urban landscape in detail, particularly concerning the inequities in cities. Second, there should be a two-pronged approach in which short-term demonstrations and their results guide and inform longer-term plans. Third, it will be crucial to unlock community potential for surveillance, innovation, education, and advocacy as well as to nudge the national governments. "This is what happened with COVID," Alabaster said. "They saw good examples of what was happening locally, and they used it to adapt and adjust their national policy."

In selling this approach to local officials, advocates should emphasize not only the value of reducing the threat of vector-borne diseases but the benefits relative to other diseases as well. "If you rethink urban space and you design it better for vector-borne diseases," he said, "there is a good chance you can also deal with the enteric diseases which are there and maybe some non-communicable diseases. . . . So, it's a win-win if we design carefully." Finally, he said, funding is always a challenge, but if short-term demonstrations can be funded, they can be used to catalyze long-term changes.

CASE STUDY FROM SINGAPORE

To illustrate some of the factors that influence arbovirus spread in an urban area, Ooi described the history of dengue incidence in Singapore. He began by showing a graph tracking the incidence of dengue versus the house index, or the percentage of houses infested with *Aedes* larvae or pupae, which is a measure of the abundance of *Aedes* mosquitoes (Figure 7-1).

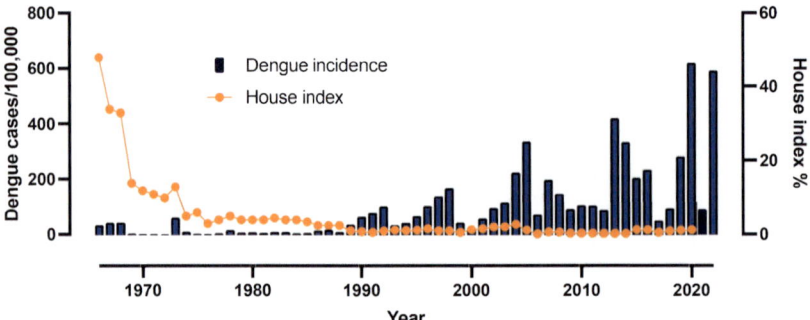

FIGURE 7-1 Dengue incidence and *Aedes* population density (house index) in Singapore, 1966–2022.
SOURCES: Presented by Eng Eong Ooi, December 13, 2023; generated with data from the Ministry of Health, Singapore.

Dengue first became a notifiable disease in Singapore in 1966, and, in response, a vector-control program was developed and implemented by K. L. Chan, the head of the Vector Control and Research branch of the Ministry of Health, which was eventually transferred to the Environment Ministry (Chan, 1985). The program began in the late 1960s with a series of studies and pilot control programs that eventually led to its formal launch in 1970. Chan described the first part of the program, which lasted until 1972, as "a loosely knitted integrated system." After a postmortem analysis of an outbreak that occurred in 1973, the vector control program was refined, and a new control strategy was developed. Still, the *Aedes aegypti* population dropped steadily beginning in 1966—before the finished vector control program was put into place—until the present. This drop in mosquitoes was likely due to the 1971 Concept Plan, developed with help from the UN Development Programme, after Singapore became an independent country in 1965. A major aspect of the plan was to free up space wherever possible, and a major opportunity for freeing up space could be found in slum housing.

In 1959, about 550,000 out of the 1.6 million people living in Singapore lived in slum housing, Ooi said. In 1960 Singapore formed the Housing Development Board to free up land by rehousing people from slum houses into high-rise apartments and to encourage home ownership. "This was partly as a way of building the nation so that the population had an ownership of the country," he said. The result was a steady decline in the number of people in slum housing to the point that by 2000, slum housing was exceptionally rare. At the same time, the number of people living in Housing Development Board flats in high-rise buildings rose dramatically, and the number of people living in high-rise condominiums that were not developed by the Housing Development Board also increased. By 1990, most of Singapore's population lived in high-rise buildings, with about 5 percent living in houses with their own land, and very few still in slums.

That transformation played a major role in the decline of the *Aedes aegypti* population in Singapore, Ooi argued. A paper published in 1971 reported on the distribution of the mosquitoes in different types of buildings in Singapore (Chan et al., 1971). It found that more than 27 percent of slum houses had mosquito larvae and that there were an average number of 5.52 larvae per housing unit. By contrast, only 5 percent of the flats in high-rise apartments had the mosquito larvae, with an average number of only 0.81 larvae per unit. A different analysis found that the *Aedes* population density in Singapore dropped sharply and then more steadily as the number of new housing units grew from 40,000 to more than 400,000 between 1966 and 1975 (Chan et al., 1985). Ooi connected the drop in mosquito population beginning in the mid-1960s to the construction on new high-rise housing, the movement of people from slum housing to the high rises, and, ultimately, the destruction of most of the slum housing.

Still, even as the amount of slum housing dropped to near zero, the population density of *Aedes aegypti* settled in at a low but non-zero level. Another factor may be playing a role in the burden of dengue in Singapore, he suggested. As the economy has steadily improved, the birth rate has steadily dropped to the point that the total fertility rate is less than two. This has led to a steady aging of the population, with the mean age of the population increasing. And that in turn, Ooi said, seems to have led to an increase in the average age and age distribution of those people in Singapore who have contracted dengue. Adult cases make up nearly 90 percent of total dengue cases in Singapore each year (Low and Ooi, 2013). This has led to a fundamental change in the type of dengue cases commonly seen in Singapore. In general, Ooi said, the rate of plasma leakage from small blood vessels is much greater in children than in adults (Gamble et al., 2000). When children are exposed to the dengue virus, they are much more likely than adults to develop dengue hemorrhagic fever, which is being characterized by plasma leakage. And, indeed, data from Singapore show that as the percentage of dengue cases that take place in those 15 years and younger has gone down, the rate of dengue hemorrhagic fever as a percentage of all cases of dengue fever has also gone down (Ooi et al., 2003). Overall, the burden of dengue has declined in Singapore, but the question still remains, however, why overall cases of dengue have increased in recent years.

The takeaway message, Ooi said, is that the rehousing of much of the Singaporean population benefited dengue prevention. Although it was motivated by economic reasons and did not involve dengue control, the change to the infrastructure seems to have significantly reduced dengue. This was combined with the changes put in motion by the growing economy, which lowered the birthrate, increased the average age of the population, and led to a lower burden of dengue hemorrhagic fever. In short, reshaping the environment has the potential to make a major difference in controlling dengue and potentially other *Aedes*-transmitted diseases.

URBAN MOSQUITO CONTROL IN AFRICA AND THE NEW MOSQUITO ON THE BLOCK

In the session's last presentation, Wilson spoke about the appearance of a new mosquito species in Africa, *Anopheles stephensi*, which carries malaria and may force those working to control malaria on the African continent to modify their strategies.

Reviewing the basics of malaria, she said it is a severe, febrile illness caused by *Plasmodium* parasites and transmitted by female *Anopheles* mosquitoes. It exerts a major public health burden, with, according to the latest World Malaria Report, a worldwide total of 249 million cases in 2022, which resulted in 608,000 deaths. In Africa, malaria is typically a rural disease, and its primary carrier is the *Anopheles gambiae* species, which likes to lay eggs in standing water such as found in puddles, ditches, and rice paddies. It typically bites humans indoors at night when they are sleeping, and it rests indoors as well. The primary control methods have been insecticide-treated bed nets and the indoor residual spraying of insecticides. These mosquito control tools, coupled with certain other effective treatments, dramatically decreased the incidence of malaria in Africa between 2000 and 2015, Wilson said, with bed nets alone being responsible for 68 percent of the decline. "This was a real success period in malaria control. However, in the past few years, we've started to see stagnation in progress and an increase in malaria cases globally, and we don't fully understand why this is."

Wilson then provided some relevant background on dengue in Africa. Dengue and other arboviral diseases have been largely neglected in Africa, she said, and for a long time, dengue has been misdiagnosed as malaria since both are febrile illnesses, and the diagnostic tools needed to distinguish between the two are often lacking. Many countries also have limited surveillance for *Aedes* mosquitoes. However, she continued, the hidden burden of dengue in Africa is becoming more widely recognized with many of the recorded outbreaks since 2011 having taken place on the eastern part of the continent.

Returning to malaria, Wilson said that in the past few years a new, invasive species of malaria-carrying mosquito, *Anopheles stephensi*, has been detected in Africa.[1] *Anopheles stephensi* is different in many ways

---

[1] During an earlier session discussion, Duane Gubler noted that the used tire trade was in fact responsible for introducing *Aedes albopictus* into the United States and Europe in the mid-1980s. He speculated that the used tire trade likely played a role in the introduction of *Aedes albopictus* into Africa as well.

from the endemic malaria mosquitoes in Africa. For instance, it is urban adapted, and it thrives in standing water in tires, water barrels, and manmade containers of the sort that *Aedes aegypti* inhabits. *Anopheles stephensi* can transmit both *Plasmodium falciparum* and *Plasmodium vivax* parasites, and it is also able to persist through dry periods with its eggs surviving for months without water. As a result, the usual seasonality seen with rural malaria in Africa is not holding for this new mosquito.

According to data from WHO, *Anopheles stephensi* is spreading across Africa (Figure 7-2). It was first identified in the Horn of Africa in Djibouti in 2012 and since then has been spreading throughout the Horn to Ethiopia, Sudan, Puntland, and Somaliland. More recently it was detected in Nigeria, Ghana, and Kenya as well, which suggested that its distribution is more widespread than originally thought. And, unfortunately, the arrival of this new species of *Anopheles* in Africa has been associated with increases in the numbers of malaria cases.

The experiences in two countries illustrate the potential dangers of this spread. Djibouti had reached pre-elimination status for malaria—the stage between control and complete elimination—in 2011, but since *Anopheles stephensi* was detected there in 2012, there has been a 36-fold increase in malaria cases. No causal connection between the arrival of *Anopheles stephensi* and the dramatic jump in malaria has been established, Wilson said, but it is "very worrying."

In Ethiopia, *Anopheles stephensi* is distributed widely throughout the country, and in 2022 there was a dry season outbreak of malaria that has been linked, at least partially, to *Anopheles stephensi* (Emiru et al., 2023). Using mathematical models, researchers at the Imperial College London have estimated that in Ethiopia *Anopheles stephensi* could cause a 50 percent increase in malaria cases, which would require an additional $72 million a year for control (Hamlet et al., 2022). Modeling studies done by Marianne Sinka from the University of Oxford suggest that an additional 126 million people in urban areas across Africa could be at risk of *Anopheles stephensi*–transmitted malaria (Sinka et al., 2020). Given the limited resources available in Africa for the control of malaria and other vector-borne diseases, she said, this situation "really presents a major threat towards effective malaria control" and elimination.

Recognizing this threat, in September 2022 WHO launched an initiative to stop the spread of *Anopheles stephensi*. Its five key components are to increase collaboration, strengthen surveillance, improve information exchange, develop guidance, and prioritize research (WHO, 2022). However, Wilson said, the initiative faces a number of challenges. *Anopheles stephensi* is difficult both to surveil and to control. The adult mosquitoes can be elusive, and there are few good traps for catching them. *Anopheles stephensi* is resistant to many of the insecticides normally used for adult

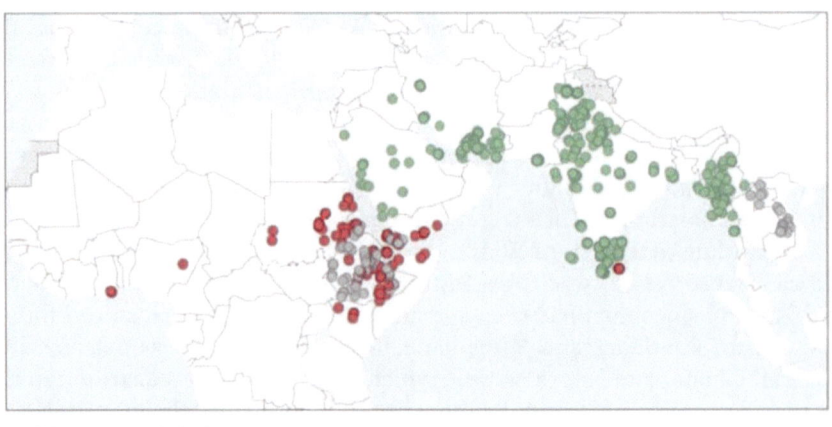

● Invasive ○ Not present ● Endemic range

FIGURE 7-2 *Anopheles stephensi* is spreading across Africa.
SOURCES: Presented by Anne Wilson, December 13, 2023. Taken from WHO Malaria Threats Map, https://apps.who.int/malaria/maps/threats/ (accessed February 24, 2024).

control. Furthermore, there is no indication that the mosquitoes engage in indoor biting or resting, so the standard malaria control tools, such as indoor residual insecticide spraying, may not work well with them. And while larval control is attractive for *Anopheles stephensi*, this approach is not widely practiced in Africa and would need capacity strengthening. Finally, there are questions about the best allocation of resources. For instance, should resources be diverted from rural malaria control programs to put more focus on cities when it is not yet clear exactly what effect *Anopheles stephensi* is likely to have on malaria incidence?

Given that *Anopheles stephensi* has commonalities with *Aedes aegypti*, Wilson said, there are opportunities for co-surveillance and co-control of the two types of mosquitoes, thereby strengthening efforts against both malaria and arboviral diseases. For instance, *Anopheles stephensi* and *Aedes aegypti* often share the same larval habitats, so there is an opportunity for integrated surveillance of both vectors as well as for integrated control by finding and removing standing water or covering water containers or using larvicides to kill the larvae.

Opportunities for synergy also exist with such things as harnessing the efforts of town councils and city leaders and engaging diverse sectors to support control and surveillance efforts for both types of mosquitoes. For example, Wilson said, several of the settings in Ethiopia where she is carrying out research on *Anopheles stephensi* suffered massive droughts, so there is no piped water. The water is brought in by private truck companies which fill household or community-owned systems of 10,000 to 20,000 liters, and these are the major habitats for the mosquitoes in these towns. "Engaging these water companies and local water sellers could be pivotal in controlling mosquitoes," she said. Finally, entire communities could be engaged in identifying and removing larval habitats. In this case, it would be important to tailor messages to the local context and explain how the presence of *Aedes aegypti* and *Anopheles stephensi* raise the risks of malaria as well as dengue and other arboviruses.

DISCUSSION

A participant began the discussion period by asking Alabaster what will be required to modify or remove slums in urban areas to limit the transmission of arboviruses.

A major problem, Alabaster replied, is that slums exist for various practical reasons, and unless there is strong political will to move forward to remove slums, they will remain. For instance, slums economically suit the slum dwellers, because many of them are single individuals who have come to a city to earn money and send that money home, and they want somewhere cheap to live. Furthermore, he continued, "many of the landlords of slum dwellers are mid-level government professionals who make a tidy living from collecting rents in slums." To get around these obstacles, it helps to have a "champion inside the ministry who is prepared to look at the long-term aspects of improving the life of those people," he said. It is also crucial to carry out a demonstration project that shows the value of the suggested changes to the community. "Once the communities are engaged, whether the mayor changes or the minister of health changes, it doesn't matter because the community will make demands from the local authority."

Lindsay, in response to a question from Lloyd, provided some additional information on the Making Cities Resilient 2030 initiative. Many organizations were involved, Lindsay said, and one of the chief drivers from the United States was the Rockefeller 100 Resilient Cities Network. When mayors from different cities get together, they are pushed by competition to do more in their own cities, and they also learn what practices have and have not worked in other areas. He noted that the initiative is not prescriptive and accounts for feasibility at the local level. Wilson added that it is important to encourage city leaders to consider vector-borne diseases as potential threats just like earthquakes, sea level rise, or long-term unemployment.

In response to an online question, Ooi said that when Singapore made the transition from slum housing to flats in high-rise apartments, it also provided piped water and improved sanitation and refuse collection. Furthermore, the fact that Singapore is a multiethnic country was considered in the transition as well, and today all of the housing estates have a mandatory ethnicity mix. "Every housing estate has to have a fair distribution of the races according to the national composition," he said, with the goal of building integrated communities.

Wilson offered a few more thoughts on combined surveillance and control efforts for both *Anopheles stephensi* and *Aedes aegypti*. There is relatively little surveillance of *Aedes* in Africa, she said, and researchers may pay attention to either *Aedes* or *Anopheles* but not both. There is a need for more coordination between these two groups to develop vector-borne disease programs instead of malaria-only programs. She noted a research group in Sudan that has an integrated vector management department that does surveillance for diseases transmitted by snails, sandflies, and mosquitoes of all sorts. Good practices do exist in some countries, she said. but they need to be expanded and strengthened.

Lloyd then directed a question about Singapore to both Ooi and Lee Ching Ng, who had spoken on the previous day. If rebuilding Singapore made such a difference in removing breeding grounds for the mosquitoes, was vector control necessary after that? Ng answered that transferring people from slums to high-rise buildings did not automatically remove the *Aedes aegypti* mosquitoes. There were still many places where water could collect, even inside the new high-rise homes. Singapore continued to educate its citizens on how to minimize the number of places that mosquitoes could breed, such as plates under a potted plant. Vector control in Singapore was focused more on removing places where standing water was available to mosquitoes rather than on such things as fogging or chemical control. Ooi added that Singapore refined its vector-control program over time to the point that it eventually became very effective.

Alabaster reiterated that the huge amount of urban space that will be built out between 2024 and 2050 offers a tremendous opportunity for creating areas where people live that are designed to resist the spread of vector-borne disease. "The incremental costs of ensuring that new urban development is future-proofed from vector-borne disease" would be minimal, he said, involving only slight changes in the design of the urban space. This new understanding of how urban design can be used to discourage the transmission of arboviruses and other vector-borne diseases is appearing at the same time as some powerful new tools, such as vaccines and environmental management, are becoming available for the prevention and control of these diseases. "So, I think the fact that the two are coming together means we have an opportunity that we shouldn't miss," he concluded.

REFERENCES

Chan, K. L. 1985. *Singapore's Dengue Haemorrhagic Fever Control Programme: A Case Study on the Successful Control of* Aedes aegypti *and* Aedes albopictus *Using Mainly Environmental Measures as Part of Integrated Vector Control*. Tokyo: SEAMIC.

Chan, Y. C., K. L. Chan, and B. C. Ho. 1971. *Aedes aegypti* (L.) and *Aedes albopictus* (Skuse) in Singapore City: 1. Distribution and density. *Bulletin of the World Health Organization* 44:617–627.

Emiru, T., D. Getachew, M. Murphy, L. Sedda, L. A. Ejigu, M. G. Bulto, I. Byrne, M. Demisse, M. Abdo, W. Chali, A. Elliott, E. N. Vickers, A. Aranda-Díaz, L. Alemayehu, S. W. Behaksera, G. Jebessa, H. Dinka, T. Tsegaye, H. Teka, S. Chibsa, P. Mumba, S. Girma, J. Hwang, M. Yoshimizu, A. Sutcliffe, H. S. Taffese, G. A. Bayissa, S. Zohdy, J. E. Tongren, C. Drakeley, B. Greenhouse, T. Bousema, and F. G .Tadesse. 2023. Evidence for a role of *Anopheles stephensi* in the spread of drug- and diagnosis-resistant malaria in Africa. *Nature Medicine* 29(12):3203–3211.

Gamble, J., D. Bethell, N. P. Day, P. P. Loc, N. H. Phu, I. B. Gartside, J. F. Farrar, and N. J. White. 2000. Age-related changes in microvascular permeability: A significant factor in the susceptibility of children to shock? *Clinical Science (London)* 98(2):211–216.

Hamlet, A., D. Dengela, J. E. Tongren, F. G. Tadesse, T. Bousema, M. Sinka, A. Seyoum, S. R. Irish, J. S. Armistead, and T. Churcher. 2022. The potential impact of *Anopheles stephensi* establishment on the transmission of *Plasmodium falciparum* in Ethiopia and prospective control measures. *BMC Medicine* 20(1):135.

Low, J. G., and E. E. Ooi. 2013. Dengue—Old disease, new challenges in an ageing population. *Annals of the Singapore Academy of Medicine* 42(8):373–375.

Ooi, E. E., K. T. Goh, and D. N. C. Wang. 2003. Effect of increasing age on the trend of dengue and dengue hemorrhagic fever in Singapore. *International Journal of Infectious Diseases* 7:231–232.

Sinka, M. E., S. Pironon, N. C. Massey, J. Longbottom, J. Hemingway, C. L. Moyes, and K. J. Willis. 2020. A new malaria vector in Africa: Predicting the expansion range of *Anopheles stephensi* and identifying the urban populations at risk. *Proceedings of the National Academy of Sciences* 117(40):24900–24908.

UNDRR (United Nations Office for Disaster Risk Reduction). n.d. MCR 2030: Making Cities Resilient. https://mcr2030.undrr.org/ (accessed February 18, 2024).

WHO (World Health Organization). 2022. *World Malaria Report 2022*. Geneva: World Health Organization. 2022. https://www.who.int/teams/global-malaria-programme/reports/world-malaria-report-2022 (accessed October 31, 2024).

World Bank. Urban Development. April 3, 2023. https://www.worldbank.org/en/topic/urbandevelopment/overview (accessed March 25, 2024).

8

Strengthening Preparedness for Arboviral Diseases

Albert I. Ko of Yale University, the moderator of the workshop's final session, said that the session's goal was to "discuss and identify the essential features of an effective, equitable, sustained multilevel response to arboviral threats—essentially, what needs to be done in the future." To that end, the session had a panel of four internationally recognized experts on arboviral diseases who work across different disciplines and regions of the world. To begin the session, each of the four panelists were asked to describe three priorities that should be included in a global response to arboviral disease. Afterwards, the panelists engaged in a moderated discussion, responding to one another's lists of priorities, and the last 30 minutes of the session was opened to questions from the audience.

PRIORITIES

The four panelists were Lee Ching Ng, Linda S. Lloyd, Audrey Lenhart of the U.S. Centers for Disease Control and Prevention, and Kariuki Njenga of Washington State University and Kenya Medial Research Institute. Several of the priorities they named shared common themes, such as collaboration and integration, the development and availability of useful tools, community engagement, environmental management, research, and funding.

Collaboration and Integration

The research and development of arboviral control measures tend to be done in isolated silos, and several of the panelists identified getting outside of these silos and working across disciplines or areas of interest as a priority.

Multiple panelists identified integrating arbovirus efforts with those aimed at other vector-borne threats as a priority. Referring to Wilson's discussion of the appearance of *Anopheles stephensi* in Africa, Lenhart noted this as a "really important opportunity where the arbovirus community could potentially leverage some of the investments that are being made in the malaria space by some of these multilateral initiatives." Because *Anopheles stephensi* breeds in locations like those preferred by *Aedes aegypti*, vector-control efforts could be made that controlled both—and thus acted against both malaria and arboviruses such as dengue.

Njenga spoke of integration more broadly. His first priority was integrating key arboviruses into the World Health Organization (WHO) African region's Integrated Disease Surveillance and Response list. "Almost all the countries follow that list," he said, and noted that very few arboviruses are currently listed. Ultimately, he said, integrating arboviruses into that system would be easier than creating a separate system to deal with arboviruses.

Ng emphasized establishing intersectoral collaborations as a priority. Singapore has the Interagency Dengue Task Force for Vector Control, which involves different national agencies and even public schools, with vector control being incorporated into the school curriculum. Singapore also has the One Health Coordinating Committee and Working Group, with five agencies that work together to design protocols and risk assessment. "I think intersectoral collaboration goes beyond just different sectors with the typical sectors that we talk about," she said. It should include, for instance, government agencies working with academia. Collaboration among field operations, laboratories, and clinicians is also valuable.

Tools

Several of the priorities mentioned involved the development and availability of effective tools for the surveillance, control, and treatment of arboviral diseases. Ng mentioned the use of replacement and suppression approaches, such as *Wolbachia* mosquitoes, as a technology that could make a major difference in Singapore, which in years past has relied on door-to-door home inspections.

Njenga offered two different types of technologies as priorities. The first was developing sustainable, affordable diagnostics for routine testing. Health departments in Africa are not testing most of their samples because the tests are inadequate, he said. Second, he called for developing and stockpiling vaccines, such as the vaccine for Rift Valley fever. There is a livestock vaccine produced in Africa, but it is just a univalent vaccine, so few farmers use it. "If we just made it multivalent so that it would be picked up by the farmers," he said, "we could be in a position to be better able to prevent Rift Valley fever," he said.

Community Engagement

Lloyd centered three of her priority actions in one area: community engagement. "I believe that if we do not have true long-term community engagement, there are no sustainable arbovirus prevention solutions," she explained, and the building of this long-term community engagement involves meeting a series of goals. The first is building trust. The second is bringing in new allies and resources. Third is creating better communication across stakeholder groups. And the fourth goal is to improve health outcomes as successful projects evolve into lasting collaborations.

Some have charged, Lloyd said, that much of what is said and written about community engagement consists mainly of vague statements and platitudes about the importance of diverse participation. She stated that the shift from such statements to true community engagement occurs by understanding more about why people do or do not do specific behaviors. Sometimes, she said, some behaviors are simply not feasible. "How do you get rid of your tires when you don't have trash collection or your trash collection service won't take them?" Other behaviors may be feasible, but they are not acceptable to the people expected to do them. "The standard scrub, rinse, and refill once a week for water storage containers is feasible," she said, "but it's not acceptable if you buy every drop of water that's used in your household, and you can't empty the container once a week." Finally, some behaviors may be both feasible and acceptable, but they are not sustainable. As an example, she pointed to illegal dumpsites in public areas. Unless the municipal government supplies the appropriate services to assist, a community cannot be expected to clean up an area repeatedly.

Next, she said, it is important to create effective strategies for building the necessary multisectoral participation to identify and implement long-term solutions that encourage and prioritize the ideas of the stakeholders. Community participation also needs to be made easier through new technologies and the selection of appropriate physical locations.

In summary, she said, community engagement approaches are needed that reflect complex urban environments and meet not just program needs but also community and individual needs. To accomplish that, she identified three priority actions:

1. Integrating community engagement for arbovirus prevention into existing initiatives such as Resilient Cities and the Healthy Cities movements;

2. Ensuring that skilled career staff lead community engagement processes that cut across ministries, organizations, and programs to sustain high levels of trust and partnership among stakeholder groups for solutions to achieve shared outcomes;
3. Funding long-term community engagement processes that focus on problem solving and achieving outcomes valued by stakeholder communities—not just those of vector-control programs.

Environmental Management

Ng described the focus on environmental management in Singapore and her belief that it should be a priority in the control of arboviruses elsewhere. Since its independence, there has been a campaign to keep Singapore clean with a focus on sanitation and hygiene. Today, people who are caught littering are fined, although she said it seems that the littering situation has gotten somewhat worse in recent decades because of the increased use of disposable items.

Environmental management also includes design modification, she said. For instance, people in Singapore high rises used to hang their clothes out to dry on a bamboo pole, but it was discovered that mosquitoes were breeding in the poles and a new design involving drying racks had to be introduced. Similarly, Singapore does not allow gutters on new buildings because they could host mosquito larvae.

Research

One of Lenhart's priorities was strengthening the evidence base for vector control. While there are some promising new tools available, there are others in development that do not yet have enough evidence accumulated to say for certain what their public health impact is and how best to use them. She called for improving the design of clinical trials of vector control tools for arboviruses. She expressed her encouragement to hear about experiences with various vaccines, particularly the chikungunya vaccine. Although there are no direct efficacy data coming out of these trials, she said, they have surrogates that track efficacy closely enough "to give us the confidence that that vaccine is a tool that can elicit a high degree of efficacy." Learning from those trials could inform how other vector-control trials are designed so that they shed light on those endpoints.

Perhaps most important in the testing of arbovirus interventions is understanding the impact of combinations of interventions, she said. "None of these things [are] ever going to be deployed in isolation," she continued, stating how preventive measures like vaccines, reactive interventions like diagnostics and therapeutics, and vector control need to be assessed collectively. Ultimately the goal should be to inform the design of context-driven, locally adapted applications of interventions.

Funding

Lenhart listed funding as another priority area that underlies all others. "We've heard about some of these promising new tools that are available, from vector control to vaccines," Lenhart said. "But then how do we bring those new tools to scale in the places that most urgently need them?" The places where interventions are most urgently needed often have significant local resource constraints. There are opportunities for multilateral initiatives. While there are several initiatives for malaria, such as the Global Fund and the U.S. President's Malaria Initiative, "there is not anything analogous in the arbovirus space," she said. There is an opportunity to convince stakeholders about the need, and in addition to the funding of programs, further research funding is also necessary. There are important gaps in needed research on vaccines, diagnostics, and therapeutics, all of which require significant research investment. Funding is needed for clinical trials for the vector-control tools, and funding research will also be important to understand the public health impacts of vector-control efforts. Finally, she said, funding decisions should consider the existing regional inequities. An example of this is the emerging situation of *Aedes*-borne arboviruses in Africa, where there is significantly less infrastructure for *Aedes* surveillance and control than elsewhere in the world.

Panel Discussion

Ko began the discussion period by asking each panelist what priorities they found particularly compelling and important to include in future responses to arboviral diseases. Ng identified Lloyd's emphasis on shaping community behavior as particularly important. She also seconded Lenhart's observation that "whatever you do, whether it's vector control or behavior change, it must be context driven; there is no 'one size fits all.'"

Lloyd highlighted Ng's point about the importance of multisectoral collaboration, including academia, clinicians, and field operations staff who are often forgotten in designing and implementing health programs. Lloyd also agreed with Lenhart about the importance of programs being context driven, adding the need for community engagement in the funding for context-driven interventions. Lenhart said that Lloyd's recommendation on community engagement is "absolutely critical" for the implementation of tools and strategies devised for arboviruses. Even with the best intervention or most efficacious tool in the world, she said, it will not matter if the community does not find it feasible, acceptable, and reasonable. Njenga identified Lenhart's point about integrating arbovirus programs into other vector-control strategies as particularly important. He also agreed with the others that community engagement will be key to ensuring the success of programs designed to prevent or control arboviral diseases.

Intersectoral Collaborations

Noting the importance of intersectoral collaborations was a theme identified by several panelists. Ko asked Lloyd whether the necessary structures exist for such partnerships and whether One Health is a viable model for such structures. Lloyd responded that it is most efficient to work within existing structures. If a country has One Health or resilient cities programs already in place, it is ideal to begin with these and build upon them.

Lenhart agreed, saying this approach is particularly important if one desires sustainability. "The bottom-up approach is the foundation for any type of sustainable intervention." Njenga added that over the past decade several changes have taken place in public health that make it easier to integrate with and build on existing systems rather than to start with entire new systems with a top-down approach. Integrating into existing systems that have been established by WHO, U.S. Centers for Disease Control and Prevention (CDC), or others and building in arbovirus surveillance and prevention should be viable in many cases, he said. Ng cautioned that the intersectoral collaboration that has been built up in Singapore may not be so easy to establish in other, larger countries. The conversations that are easy to have in Singapore may be much more difficult in other places.

Vector Control

Noting "broad enthusiasm" among the panelists for vector control being a key component of controlling arboviral diseases, Ko asked how to balance the need for evidence with the desire to move forward quickly and save lives. "We're really in an unprecedented time where there is a lot of innovation around vector control, especially for the *Aedes*-borne arboviruses," Lenhart said. "But the piece that is missing to a certain extent is understanding what works best under what circumstances and where." A particular technique may be a major success story in one setting but yield much less impressive results somewhere else, and understanding why that is the case is important so policy makers in different countries have the best evidence at their disposal when they are determining where to spend their limited funds for vector control. This is where implementation science is valuable, she continued, and understanding the types of settings where people will be receptive to certain interventions.

Ko followed up by asking about the value of randomized controlled trials (RCT) versus studies with quasi-experimental designs. "RCTs are an incredibly powerful tool for helping us to understand what the public health impact of these tools are," Lenhard replied, but noted that other trial designs are important and there is much to learn in terms of possibilities with modeling and how this can inform vector-control tools.

Noting that RCTs can be expensive, Ng suggested making it a requirement to prove a method through an RCT could hold new innovations back. She noted the importance of more innovative evaluations for vector-control tools, such as data analytics and synthetic controls.

Lloyd added that RCTs are not amenable to looking at how communities interact with a technology and then what happens over time. "We don't have variables for how people interact with these technologies," she said. "There are no variables. We have to create them and validate them, and I think that there are other frameworks that we can use."

Surveillance

Responding to a question from Ko about surveillance, Ng said it is important to recognize that different types of surveillance are needed in different countries. In the case of dengue, the disease is endemic in some countries and emerging in others, while others are trying to keep dengue out. Each of them will need a different surveillance strategy. Some countries will require comprehensive surveillance, for instance, while others may only need sentinel surveillance in hospitals and health care clinics. Whatever the requirements, those in charge of surveillance should be familiar with the patterns of arbovirus outbreaks in their countries and in nearby areas.

Njenga said that there is a movement in Africa to go from indicator-based surveillance, which WHO has relied on for many years, to event-based surveillance, a shift that is being driven by the U.S. Agency for International Development and CDC. Event-based surveillance, which is being pilot tested in several countries, is community-driven, relying on individuals in the community to report suspected cases. It is intended to spot likely cases earlier than is possible when relying on hospitals to detect and report cases, and it has potential to vastly improve detection in resource-limited areas that cannot afford expensive surveillance systems, Njenga said. What needs improvement is the availability of tests that can detect the presence of arboviruses in suspected cases. Lloyd said that data presentation is critical regardless of the surveillance system. Data must be presented differently depending on the purpose, such as justifying a surveillance program to managers or communicating a risk to a community.

Equity

Inequity can be minimized by working with the existing systems, Njenga said. As an example, he pointed to the Africa CDC, which he said has "completely transformed" outbreak response and advocacy for Africa. It has been so successful, he said, because it was integrated under the preexisting African Union, which facilitated rapid buy-in from African countries and led to reduced inequity. Countries like Singapore are likely to always be better than most in their control of arboviruses, Njenga said, but it is possible to make sure that low- and middle-income countries will not be too far behind in the case of a major epidemic. "Maybe they are one step behind, but not five steps behind, as has happened in the past," he said.

Lloyd said that one factor in ensuring equity in arbovirus control and prevention will be creating equity in access to water and sanitation. "It's really hard to ask people to do things when they don't have clean water, when they don't have sanitation, when they have dirt roads that collect water." Lenhart continued along the same lines. "I think inequity is embedded in the fabric of all of this," she said, "because at the end of the day, these diseases disproportionately affect the poorest in the world." Context-driven, locally adapted solutions will account for various drivers behind the disease outbreaks and the role that poverty plays. She added that one of the challenges in addressing arboviral diseases is that there are always competing health priorities, and arboviruses do not kill people on the same scale as diseases like malaria. "It's not to minimize the impact that the arboviruses have," she said. "It's just, in realistic terms, that's what's being faced."

Vaccines

Ko asked the panelists about the role of arbovirus vaccines in the future. Lloyd responded that vaccines are another tool that needs to be reviewed on a country level and assessed based on acceptability and feasibility at a local level. Ng said she believes that once a safe, effective vaccine is developed and tested, there will be countries that use it. However, there are questions related to the use of vaccines against arboviruses, such as the role of cross-reactivity. In general, a vaccine designed for a particular virus, such as dengue, will not protect against others, such as Zika and chikungunya. Thus, arbovirus protection will likely require multiple vaccines. "That's why I think vector control is very important," she said. "It solves three problems in one go."

Njenga said that vaccines do have an important role to play and pointed to Rift Valley fever as an example. It is seen mostly in Africa and affects domesticated animals such as cattle but can also jump into humans. Livestock vaccines exist, and if it were possible to get to the point where livestock were routinely vaccinated, he said, it would reduce the risk of a major epidemic of Rift Valley fever to near zero. The uptake of the vaccine by farmers has so far been relatively low, but there has been an effort to create a multivalent vaccine that would protect livestock against Rift Valley fever along with other diseases that are more concerning to farmers. If that effort succeeds, Njenga said, it will instantly make Rift Valley fever a limited problem. Lenhart said that vaccines are critically important and should be part of an integrated strategy for arboviral disease control, which would also include vector control. Thus, further research and development of vaccines should take place to improve this aspect of the toolbox.

QUESTION-AND-ANSWER PERIOD

Peter Daszak, president of EcoHealth Alliance, opened the question-and-answer period with a question about detecting emerging diseases. He asked why diagnosing febrile illness is so difficult in various countries, as Njenga had described.

Njenga responded that there are many accurate diagnostic tests for arboviruses that are simply not available in low- and middle-income countries. "[This is] an embarrassing statement to make for viruses that we have had for centuries. . . . Why can't we work to make diagnostics a bit more sustainably and affordably available?" However, he added that some of the most advanced technologies, such as genomics tests and rapid sequencing, are beginning to appear in Africa, thanks to the work done in response to the COVID-19 pandemic. These advancements will make it possible to come up with diagnoses that could not be made before.

An audience member, Randy Nett of the CDC commented on a point that had been made the day before by Erin Staples and Peter Hotez about the lack of uniformity of vector control and vector surveillance in the United States. He noted it will be important to have vector control in every community and make sure that it is a systematic operation with a basic set of abilities and practices. In this respect, Ko commented, the United States could learn from countries in the Global South, particularly Brazil, "where they have zoonotic control centers of the highest quality that can react to rabies, yellow fever, recurrent leptospirosis, everything, in addition to dengue, Zika, and so forth."

Next, Matthew Zahn, who works in local public health in Orange County, Southern California, made a comment about the difficulties of vector control and prevention in the United States. In his county of 3 million people, which he described as the sixth largest county in the United States, there is a vector-control program that conducts surveillance, but it is up to the public health entity to respond when a vector of potential risk is detected. Unfortunately, he continued, the decision about what to do is often a political one, and the politicians are likely to fall back on responses that individuals can do—or choose not to do—on their own. He noted public acceptance is a challenge for interventions such as *Wolbachia*-infected mosquitoes, even if only from a small minority.

A virtual attendee suggested that socioeconomic issues need to be considered as part of any arbovirus strategy, saying that the disease risk can be stratified using these considerations to better determine whether to take preventive and reactive interventions in different locations or contexts. Lenhart agreed with a virtual comment that socioeconomic issues need to be considered as part of an arbovirus strategy and can be used to stratify disease risks. She added that there are close associations between certain sociodemographic factors and risk of arboviral diseases. Traditionally, she added, analyses of disease hotspots have looked predominantly at historic patterns of disease transmission, but incorporating some socioeconomic factors could "perhaps further refine those types of predictive models."

Concerning prediction, Anne Wilson, a presenter in the previous session, asked, "what are some of the things that we can do to be prepared for anything?" Valerie Paz-Soldán of Tulane University suggested that community engagement could be important as long as effective systems existed for collecting and disseminating data. These systems should not only be user-friendly in terms of collecting data so that everyone can use them, but also should have some sort of dashboard function that easily allows community members to see the status of their community. Too often, she said, data from low- and middle-income countries go to the country's health ministry or the Pan American Health Organization (PAHO) or a similar organization, "and unless somebody is really curious and looks at the report, they just won't know what happened with all that information." Thais dos Santos of PAHO noted that the most effective way to engage with communities is by using their own evidence. As PAHO has seen with some of its own programs, people in communities get motivated by seeing "the actual impact of their own actions."

9

Closing Remarks

Each of the workshop's two days ended with a brief session summarizing that day's remarks. The summaries offered a chance to look back on the high points of the workshop.

DAY 1: CURRENT LANDSCAPE AND RISK ASSESSMENT OF ARBOVIRAL THREATS

Peter Daszak of EcoHealth Alliance summarized the first day's proceedings.

In his introductory remarks, Thomas W. Scott focused on the complexity of arbovirus life cycles and the drivers of disease risk, which create challenges for surveillance, control, and mitigation techniques. However, Daszak noted, "complexity drives innovation," which should eventually lead to answers.

Next, Eve Lackritz spoke about the Zika roadmap. Her talk, Daszak said, was "a reminder of where we are and what we don't have yet despite decades of research." For Zika, that means no vaccines, no diagnostics, and no antenatal tests. "It is a disgrace," he said, "that such a devastating disease leaves us 10 years on with this situation."

The first panel, with speakers Duane Gubler, Sylvain Aldighieri, Laura Kramer, and Raman Velayudhan, described the current situation with arboviruses. A major message there, Daszak said, is that complacency is a problem. New arbovirus outbreaks will continue occurring, yet not enough is being done to prepare for them. The session also covered the underlying drivers of arboviral disease, such as population growth, urbanization, global travel, and global climate change. Various comments indicated the seriousness of the arboviral threat, including how the West Nile virus expanded in the United States and the fact that there is local transmission of dengue in places like Arizona, California, Texas, and Florida as well as France, Italy, and Portugal.

The second session, with speakers Diana Rojas, Nuno Faria, Lee Ching Ng, and Debi Boeras (speaking for Rosanna Peeling), described several positive developments in epidemiological surveillance, genomic surveillance, risk assessment, and diagnostics. For instance, genomics and hotspot mapping can be used to better target surveillance to the places that most need it. Ng's case study of Singapore shows what is possible with an integrated combination of various techniques, including rapid testing and community alerts and a carrot-and-stick approach to individual compliance.

The third session focused on different ways to combat arboviral threats, including vaccines, vector control, surveillance, and modeling. The speakers were Gabriela Paz-Bailey, Thomas W. Scott, Thais dos Santos, and Oliver Brady. One clear message, Daszak said, is that the complexity of arboviral diseases is a challenge to finding effective responses. Particularly striking, he said, is how slow progress is on vaccines. Although there have been some developments in chikungunya, yellow fever, and dengue, vaccines are still a work in progress for Zika and West Nile, he added Among the challenges are how sporadic the outbreaks are, the complexity of the life cycles, and the uncertainty of the market. Some good news is that targeted residential spraying led to a 90 percent reduction in dengue cases in Australia. "These interventions work," Daszak said, but what is lacking is the implementation science, such as trials of single and multiple interventions. "That is happening now, and it's really quite an exciting time." The experience of the Pan American Health Organization (PAHO) with virtual collaborative spaces shows how hard it is to work with different countries and share data in a rapid way. Although the idea of virtual collaborative might seem obvious to some, Daszak noted the large amount of work that has been invested to gain trust from countries to allow rapid information sharing for diseases of public health relevance.

The day's final session had Erin Staples and Peter Hotez speaking on lessons learned from previous outbreaks. Daszak found two phrases particularly memorable: Staples's reference to having "an arbovirologist in every state," and Hotez's phrase of "arbovirus tsunami" as the sort of language that people in the room should be using to get better funding and more recognition for these diseases.

DAY 2: INNOVATION FOR FUTURE ARBOVIRUS MITIGATION

Thomas W. Scott, Distinguished Professor at University of California, Davis, offered a summary of the second day. He began with Session five, whose speakers were Jamie Lloyd-Smith, Nikos Vasilakis, Segaran Pillai, and Valerie Paz-Soldán. One of the topics was analytical tools, which can be used, for example, to understand animal-to-human transmission. Such transmission requires a series of critical steps for a virus to spread, and these can be used to identify viruses of greatest concern and to tease apart the elements of spillover, which might lead to targets for intervention. Vasilakis spoke about mechanisms to assimilate, interpret, and implement data with the goal of identifying the drivers behind virus emergence and spread to better understand how to interfere with outbreaks. Pillai discussed how to rank different viruses according to their risk. This makes it possible to stratify viruses by the degree of health concern. Then Paz-Soldán spoke about implementation and the behavioral and social sciences and argued that when one is assessing the public health value of a tool, it is critical to look at the details associated with the real-world implementation of that tool. Scott said that this brings up the crucial difference between the efficacy and effectiveness of an intervention. Efficacy is how well the intervention works in perfectly controlled circumstances and can be judged best through randomized controlled trials (RCTs). Effectiveness, on the other hand, is what happens in the real world. This is a critical point, Scott said, because one can have amazing RCT results that indicate an intervention is very promising, but "if we don't know how to implement it and we don't do it correctly, we're not going to get the outcome that we want." He suggested that effective use has been a problem with many of the tools that have been developed over the past 50–70 years.

Session six, with speakers Steven Lindsay, Graham Alabaster, Eng Eong Ooi, and Anne Wilson, was devoted to the urban environment and how best to manage it. Lindsay described the concept of "building *Aedes* out," which suggests that new urban development and construction should be carried out in a way that minimizes the transmission of viruses by mosquitoes. Scott described this as "a city-led, locally adapted new paradigm for proactive urban viral disease prevention." Lindsay also spoke about linking arboviral disease prevention with networks like Resilient Cities or Healthy Cities, Healthy People. There are people already moving forward with these networks, Scott said, but arboviruses are not on their radar. "So, it's really up to us to engage with them and get them to start thinking about how they could benefit if they included this in what they're doing."

Alabaster spoke about how urban expansion is an opportunity for local public health improvement, such as can be accomplished by things like solid waste removal, which would improve the quality of people's lives but also reduce the breeding sites for *Aedes aegypti*. That in turn can mobilize local support for more of such efforts and their long-term maintenance. The two-pronged approach that Alabaster described can be a very powerful tool. To get political support for a project, Scott said, one cannot have a program that goes beyond election cycles and takes 10 to 20 years to show results. A better approach, he continued, is to do a short-term project on a limited scale, and apply the best tools, and then use the positive results from the program to build support for a larger, longer-term program.

Of all the techniques available right now, Scott said, one of the most promising is targeted indoor residual spraying along with larval control. At the same time, there should be an effort to push new construction in a direction that will make it easier to disrupt the transmission of arboviruses, he continued. Vector control will always be necessary, he said, but if new development and construction is done in a way that accounts for virus transmission, future efforts may rely less on direct vector control and more on the built environment. Singapore, as discussed by Ooi, offers a case study of how reshaping the built environment in innovative ways can have a major effect on arboviral transmission as well as on the standard of living in an area. Wilson made the case that, with the appearance of *Anopheles stephensi* mosquitoes, there is an opportunity for synergy between malaria control efforts and arboviral control efforts.

Finally, Scott reviewed the workshop's final session, which captured the most important aspects identified in the workshop for strengthening preparedness for arboviral diseases. The speakers/discussants in that session were Lee Ching Ng, Linda S. Lloyd, Audrey Lenhart, and Kariuki Njenga.

One question that arose in the session was whether RCTs are necessary. They can have a real benefit, Scott said, pointing to the remarkable RCT result against dengue for the vector-control method using *Wolbachia* replacements. On the other hand, he said, there are clearly issues with effectiveness versus efficacy, and it can be very difficult to carry out RCTs with multiple different implementation arms. A key message from the session was the importance of community engagement if a program is to be sustainable, including having the right leaders in place in the community. As such, the chosen location to do a pilot study can make all the difference.

Scott shared that four other major themes that emerged were the value of context-driven, socially adapted interventions; the importance of funding effectiveness trials; the opportunity offered by projects that address arboviruses at the same time as they address other disease; and the need to strengthen the evidence base. The experience in Singapore shows that a very effective vector-control program can result in lower herd immunity of a population to the point that an outbreak is possible even when there are very few mosquitoes. Thus, Scott said, "Vector control unto itself is not sustainable for the long-term. It can have an effect for a period of time, but a long-term sustainable intervention should combine different strategies, he said.

Speaking of points of interest from the workshop, Scott named the work done by Lloyd-Smith on modeling zoonotic spillover, noting the importance of taking a systematic approach to understanding the processes that are involved to prevent disease. He also highlighted Pillai's systematic ranking of risks as a way of targeting interventions and Njenga's discussion of how getting a multivalent vaccine for domestic animals could almost eliminate epidemic Rift Valley fever transmission. He also noted Steven Lindsay's comments on the importance of the built environment and demonstrating benefits of environmental management to city leaders to gain buy-in and enact sustainable change.

Scott highlighted one take-home message for workshop attendees: if the status quo of inaction prevails, the situation will only become worse. The workshop has provided insight on ways to move forward with innovative and integrated arbovirus control, and action must be taken to apply these strategies to make meaningful progress.

A

Workshop Statement of Task

Mitigating Arboviral Threats and Strengthening Public Health Preparedness: A Workshop

December 12-13, 2023, Washington, DC

PURPOSE

A planning committee of the National Academies of Sciences, Engineering, and Medicine will organize a public workshop to explore the role of arbovirus mitigation within the context of public health preparedness and capacity building. Workshop discussions will consider potential actions that can be taken to understand and mitigate arboviral disease threats and highlight priority areas for research and investment through examining:

1. Lessons learned from Zika and chikungunya epidemics, including shared learnings from COVID-19 and mpox;
2. Aspects of public health preparedness, such as environmental and urban planning issues, that will mutually benefit from enhanced arbovirus mitigation;
3. Current efforts and approaches for determining high-risk pathogens and vectors;
4. Current capacity for detecting, diagnosing, and scaling up testing for exotic arboviruses (including surveillance systems and diagnostic laboratory capacity);

5. The status of vaccine development and availability for arboviruses, including highlights of promising technologies for advancement;
6. Development and use of vector-targeted mitigation and elimination strategies, including the current status and potential impact of innovative technologies; and
7. Strategies for strengthening and supporting the necessary workforce in research, development, and public health to address arboviral threats.

The planning committee will organize the workshop, develop the agenda, select speakers and discussants, and moderate or identify moderators for the discussions. A proceedings publication that summarizes the presentations and discussions held during this workshop will be prepared by a designated rapporteur in accordance with institutional guidelines.

B

Public Meeting Agenda

MITIGATING ARBOVIRAL THREATS AND STRENGTHENING
PUBLIC HEALTH PREPAREDNESS: A WORKSHOP

Virtual webcast or at the National Academy of Sciences
2101 Constitution Ave., NW, Washington, D.C. | Lecture Room

Day 1: December 12, 2023 (9:00 AM ET – 5:00 PM ET)

9:00 AM ET	**Welcome remarks, workshop overview, and goals** Peter Daszak (EcoHealth Alliance), *Workshop Co-chair* *Chair, Forum on Microbial Threats* Thomas W. Scott (University of California, Davis), *Workshop Co-chair*
9:15 – 11:15 AM ET	**Advancing global arbovirus research priorities** Eve Lackritz (CIDRAP)
9:45 – 11:15 AM ET	**Session 1: Current and Emerging Threats from Arboviral Disease—Burden and Future Risk** Marcos Espinal (PAHO) *Session Moderator*

	Duane Gubler (Duke National University of Singapore)
	Sylvain Aldighieri (PAHO)
	Laura Kramer (State University of New York at Albany)
	Raman Velayudhan (WHO)
11:15 – 11:30 AM ET	**BREAK**
11:30 – 1:00 PM ET	**Session 2: Assessing and Detecting Arboviral Risk**
	Eva Harris (University of California, Berkeley)
	Session Moderator
	Diana Rojas (WHO)
	Nuno Faria (Imperial College London)
	Lee Ching Ng (Environmental Health Institute Singapore)
	Rosanna Peeling (London School of Hygiene and Tropical Medicine)
1:00 – 2:00 PM ET	**LUNCH**
2:00 – 3:30 PM ET	**Session 3: Response to Arboviral Threats**
	Ann Powers (CDC)
	Session Moderator
	Gabriela Paz-Bailey (CDC)
	Thomas W. Scott (University of California, Davis)
	Thais dos Santos (PAHO)
	Oliver Brady (London School of Hygiene and Tropical Medicine)
3:30 – 3:45 PM ET	**BREAK**
3:45 – 4:45 PM ET	**Session 4: Lessons Learned from Previous Outbreaks**
	Kent Kester (IAVI)
	Session Moderator
	Erin Staples (CDC)
	Peter Hotez (Baylor College of Medicine)

4:45 – 5:00 PM ET	**Synthesis and adjourn** Peter Daszak (EcoHealth Alliance) *Workshop Co-chair* *Chair, Forum on Microbial Threats*

Day 2: December 13, 2023 (9:00 AM ET – 3:15 PM ET)

9:00 AM ET	**Welcome remarks, review of day 1** Peter Daszak (EcoHealth Alliance), *Workshop Co-chair* *Chair, Forum on Microbial Threats*
9:15 – 10:45 AM ET	**Session 5: Arbovirus Spillover and Spread** Peter Daszak (EcoHealth Alliance) *Session Moderator* Jamie Lloyd-Smith (University of California, Los Angeles) Nikos Vasilakis (University of Texas Medical Branch) Segaran Pillai (Food and Drug Administration) Valerie Paz-Soldán (Tulane University)
10:45 – 11:00 AM ET	**BREAK**
11:00 – 12:30 PM ET	**Session 6: Urban Development and Management** Linda Lloyd (San Diego State University) *Session Moderator* Steven Lindsay (Durham University) Graham Alabaster (UN Habitat) Eng Eong Ooi (Duke National University of Singapore) Anne Wilson (Liverpool School of Tropical Medicine)
12:30 – 1:30 PM ET	**LUNCH**
1:30 – 3:00 PM ET	**Session 7: Strengthening Preparedness for Arboviral Diseases** Albert Ko (Yale University) *Session Moderator* Lee Ching Ng (Environmental Health Institute of Singapore) Linda Lloyd (San Diego State University)

Audrey Lenhart (CDC)
Kariuki Njenga (Washington State University)

3:00 – 3:15 PM ET **Synthesis and close**
Thomas W. Scott (University of California-Davis)
Workshop Co-chair